"Caregiver Success"
CAREGIVER SUCCESS: TIPS AND TOOLS

"Nancy the Nurse Practitioner's" tips and medical guidelines to empower success for the aging or disabled person and the caregiver

ANN (NANCY) RHODES, APRN-BC

Copyright © 2024 Ann (Nancy) Rhodes, APRN-BC.

All rights reserved. No part of this book may be reproduced, stored, or transmitted by any means—whether auditory, graphic, mechanical, or electronic—without written permission of both publisher and author, except in the case of brief excerpts used in critical articles and reviews. Unauthorized reproduction of any part of this work is illegal and is punishable by law.

ISBN: 979-8-89419-170-6 (sc)
ISBN: 979-8-89419-171-3 (hc)
ISBN: 979-8-89419-172-0 (e)

Because of the dynamic nature of the Internet, any web addresses or links contained in this book may have changed since publication and may no longer be valid. The views expressed in this work are solely those of the author and do not necessarily reflect the views of the publisher, and the publisher hereby disclaims any responsibility for them.

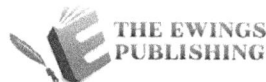

One Galleria Blvd., Suite 1900, Metairie, LA 70001
(504) 702-6708

Contents

Introduction 1
Preface. 3
Disclaimer 5
A Prayer for the Caregiver 6
Dedication. 7
The Hummingbird. 9
What does Compassion Mean? 11
Being an Advocate for You and your Loved One 13
What is a Nurse Practitioner? 15

Section I: Tips and Tools to Care for the Older Adult/Disabled

Who are We Caring for? Why Should We Look our Best?. 21
Finding Your Purpose as an Older Adult 23
Taking Care of the Caregiver. 25
Get Connected 32
Get Organized 34
Your Aide. 38
What is Cultural Diversity?. 42
The Art of Listening 43
Advanced Care Planning 46
Ageism. 47
The Annual Wellness Exam 48
Burial and Funeral Plans- are you prepared? 51
The Bedridden Patient 54
    How to make a bed with someone in it (an occupied bed) 54
        How to position someone in bed 55

How to pull someone up in bed. 57
How to change an undergarment in bed. 58
How to wash someone's hair in bed. 59
How to give someone a bath in bed 60
How To Use a Hoyer Lift 61
Stimulation for the bedridden patient 64
Change can be good 65
Durable Medical Equipment- What is it? (DME). 67
Elder and Caregiver Abuse 70
Fall Prevention. 71
Fire Prevention: What to do in Case of a Fire 78
Hand Washing/ Nail Care. 80
Heat Safety Tips 82
How to Take Vital Signs. 83
Humor and Introspection- Time to laugh. 89
Hurricane Safety Tips 90
Long-Term Care Insurance- Have you considered it?. 91
Money Matters- What is a Personal Money Manager? 93
Mouth Care. 95
The Healing Power Music has on Seniors. 99
Pets- what they mean to us 100
Podiatry-Having a Professional Take Care of your Feet 102
What is a Prosthetist/ Orthotist? 103
Power Outage- Be Prepared! 104
Rehabilitation. 105
How to Care for your Respiratory Equipment 110
How to Use and Take Care of Your Nebulizer 110
How to Use/ How to take care of oxygen equipment
(Oxygen Concentrators/ Nasal Cannula) 112
How to assemble a new portable cylinder 114
How to apply a nasal cannula tubing 115
How to Use/ care for your/BIPAP, CPAP machine 116

Safety tips while on oxygen therapy 118
Safe Storage and Disposal of Medications 119
Saving Energy When You Have a Chronic Condition .120
Social Workers- What can they do for you? 125
Spirituality - Finding your peace, and how faith gives you hope 126
How to use/ Care for your Portable Suction Machine 127
Telehealth 129
Tornado Safety Tips 130
Transportation 131
"Upsizing" Your Home 132
You Can Stop Smoking 136
Winter Safety Tips 140

Section II: Medical Conditions of the Older Adult

Anemia 145
Arthritis- osteoarthritis or rheumatoid 146
Aspiration- How to Prevent it 148
Atrial Fibrillation (AF)- what exactly is this? 151
Cancer in the Older Adult 153
Congestive Heart Failure (CHF) 154
Constipation 158
Deep Vein Thrombosis (DVT) -What is it and how to you prevent it? 161
Dehydration- What should you watch for? 166
The Aging Brain 169
Types of Dementia 170
Diabetes Mellitus 175
Eating Right for Older Adults 179
Eye care and complications 192
Foot Care Guidelines for Everyone especially over 60 198
Fractures 205
Fungal Dermatitis (Candidal Intertrigo) 207

Gastrostomy Tube- having one inserted (G-Tube). 210
Hard of Hearing- Is it wax?? 212
Head Injury 213
Hypercholesterolemia- Do you need to be on a statin at 90? 216
Hypertension 219
 How to take a blood pressure reading. 221
Lung Disorders 224
Lymphedema. 228
Medication Tips. 229
Mental Health Conditions 234
Obesity in the Older Adult 244
Osteoporosis- what it is and how to prevent it. 246
Oxygen Deprivation 251
Pain- How do you manage it? 253
Palliative Care-what is it? 263
Parkinson's Disease. 264
Pneumonia 267
Probiotics- how do they help the gut?. 270
Restless Legs Syndrome (RLS) 271
Skin Conditions and Care 272
 Preventing Skin Tears. 272
 Skin Breakdowns: How does a pressure ulcer occur? 276
 Skin Conditions 292
 How to prevent skin cancer:. 295
Sleep Problems (Insomnia) 303
Sprains and Strains 306
Stomach Problems. 308
 Leaky Gut- what is that??. 309
 Heartburn- understanding how to treat it. 311
 Nausea and Vomiting 314
 Appendicitis. 315
 Diverticulitis. 315
 Hernia- what is it?. 317

Stroke- What is it and what are the symptoms 318
    What is a TIA? 320
Syncope (Fainting Episode) 321
Thyroid Disease. 323
Upper Respiratory Infection 325
Urinary Tract Conditions. 328
Urinary Tract Infection (UTI). 330
How to Collect a Urine Specimen
    Continent Male. 333
    Incontinent Male 334
    Continent Female 335
    Incontinent Female 337
What other types of catheters are there? 340
Prevention of Urinary Tract Infection (UTI) 341
Acute Urinary Retention 344
Benign Prostatic Hypertrophy or Hyperplasia (BPH) 345
Vaccines 346
Vaginal Yeast Infection 349
When We Reach the End of Our Lives- 350
The Five Stages of Grief 355
What is Ambiguous Loss? 357
Moving on.... the next chapter for the caregiver 359
Epilogue. 361
The Glossary 363

Introduction

The purpose of this book is to help you, the caregiver, to learn helpful tips so you can take care of someone; and hopefully, prevent unnecessary suffering and hospitalizations. These ideas are a conglomerate of years of experience and thought, both taken from evidence-based information and good old common sense from the insight of a nurse practitioner and from creative caregivers. As the baby boomer ages (which is 10,000 a day until the year 2030), I thought, who is going to take care of us?

At any time, our lives could change in an instant and we are now a full-time caregiver. Perhaps someone we love suffers from a stroke, a debilitating fall, or we have a child with cancer.

This book also provides guidance for the caregiver to prevent caregiver stress and burn-out by emphasizing the need to fulfill our physical, mental and spiritual well-being.

Hello, my name is Ann Rhodes and known by many of my patients and colleagues as Nancy. Just call me "Nancy the Nurse Practitioner!"

I am an influencer on my YouTube channel, "Caregiver Success" where you can see practical videos for care and many more that are inspirational as well as spiritual. Please subscribe and leave comments so I can get to know you. Thank you for taking this caregiving journey with me.

Preface

This book was supposed to exist. After years of gathered thoughts and ideas about caregiving, it was imperative that I sit down and organize this learning tool. I had a box full of memoirs: letters from patients, Christmas cards, tons of ideas from funny to very serious, that I thought were needed to be mentioned here, in order to be a successful caregiver.

I want to thank all my patients who allowed and entrusted me to come into their homes and their lives. We had many meaningful times together- good and sad. I also thank you for consenting to have your faces and experiences in the book so others could learn and feel secure caring for someone.

Disclaimer

All pictures of patients and caregivers provided written permission to the author to use them in this book. The information in this book has been taken from many sources and teaching aids, and highlights many studies, including my personal views.

As you know, due to ongoing findings in the area of medicine, this information may not cover all recent changes and findings. This information is not all-inclusive, nor is this book intended to be a substitute for professional medical advice, diagnosis, or treatment.

The Author cannot be responsible for any damages due to the information presented in this book. All photographs are the property of the Author as are real stories and anecdotes that helped the Author envision the need for this book. Medical equipment and items mentioned are used for the sole reason to guide with solutions to care and by trademarks, trade names, model numbers, etc., by their owners.

A Prayer for the Caregiver

Dear Lord,

I pray that you will give strength and patience to the caregiver as they care for their loved ones.

That you provide emotional health to him/her showing peace and resilience in order to deal with stress and anxiety.

I pray for their physical well-being asking for restful sleep, and good health so they can carry out their responsibilities.

And, please, Lord, provide wisdom so that they can make good decisions.

With your guidance, I pray that family and friends as well as the community surrounds them with support.

Lastly, oh Lord, and most importantly, I pray that the caregiver shows compassion and empathy towards themselves and their loved ones. In your name, Amen.

Dedication

I dedicate this, my first book, to God, and to my mom and dad. You raised me with humor, tenacity, compassion and most of all, the love of people. To my husband, Steve who has been very supportive, and to my son Travis, and my daughter, Chelsea; and most of all to you, the caregiver who gives so much each day, unselfishly. I hope this book provides many of the answers to help you care for someone in your life.

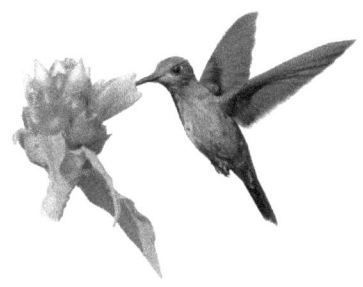

The Hummingbird

The story about the hummingbird comes from an experience I had one year to the day my father-in-law died - August 31, 2017.

I was working on this book at the time, and as I was going through the manuscript, a hummingbird appeared at my window. It was buzzing busily at my window for a long time and seemed to be looking at me. When I looked up, he flew away.

Later in the day, I was in our vegetable garden picking beans and cucumbers. I could hear a soft buzzing in my ear, and as I looked up there was the hummingbird. I put down the bowl of vegetables and began to talk to the hummingbird. He seemed to be listening staying near for a long time. I had a sense of peace and joy and felt Dad's presence. What a blessing that was!

In Native American culture, hummingbirds are seen as healers and bringers of love, good luck, and joy. They are a reminder that our happiness lies within us.

In addition, when a loved one has passed on, the hummingbird may be a sign that they have successfully made it to the other side and is doing just fine. The hummingbird became my book logo!

What does Compassion Mean?

What does the word, compassion, mean to you? Do you think you are a compassionate person? Being a caregiver is a tremendous undertaking. Be honest with yourself. If you do not feel you can take care of the person, make other arrangements. Some people are not meant to be caregivers. Give yourself grace and do not feel guilty about it!

But if you are ready to perform this role you are now a caregiver! You could be the daughter of an older parent, or an older spouse; you could be caring for a disabled child, working as an aide, a nursing student, or anyone in healthcare, etc. We are all caregivers at one time or another and throughout our lives.

According to Strauss et al. (2016), the 5 elements of compassion are:

1. recognizing suffering
2. understanding of the existence of suffering in the human experience
3. having feeling for the person who is suffering and feeling emotionally connected
4. tolerating any feelings you may be feeling, even if uncomfortable
5. motivation to act/ acting to alleviate suffering

Empathy and compassion are not the same. Empathy is where you actually feel the other person's emotional pain. Compassion, on the other hand, is when you take action to help the other person. The latter is what a caregiver does every minute of every day caring for someone.

Compassion, at the core of it, is about putting aside any judgement and refusing to turn away from a situation that is challenging. It requires you to suffer along with the person you are caring for. The feeling actually arises in you when you are confronted with another person's suffering.

It is important to know that compassion promotes meaningful connections, aids in problem-solving and improves one's health and wellbeing. It has been found that a compassionate workplace culture reduces burnout and actually increases productivity by 12% or more.

Here are some ways you can show compassion to others:

- Speak with kindness
- Apologize when you have made a mistake
- Listen carefully and without judgment
- Be encouraging
- Be helpful
- Be happy for someone else's success
- Be non-judgmental

In the book called "Holy Moments" by Matthew Kelly, he speaks repeatedly about random acts of kindness. We have all experienced it. A stranger in front of you on a coffee line buys your coffee, or a present arrives at your door from a neighbor for no reason. Are you one of those people that performs holy moments? You can be!

<blockquote>The bottom line is to follow the Golden Rule:
"Do unto others as you would have them do unto you."</blockquote>

As you read through this book, full of stories, procedures and medical conditions, learn to incorporate compassion in everything, and you will gain a feeling of purpose and wellbeing. Just imagine how the world would be if we all practiced "holy moments?"

Being an Advocate for You and your Loved One

My husband, Steve, just had his hip replaced. But before he did, he explored many surgeons who were in his insurance plan. He then checked their credentials, how many surgeries of this kind he had performed and he checked with his insurance about extraneous costs he may incur.

In the meantime, I found a lending company to get a walker and a cane to borrow so we did not have to purchase them. We went to the pharmacy to get the 5 medications he would be taking post-surgery. Two of them were expensive, so we checked some drug discount programs- Single care and Array Rx getting the costs down from 200.00 to 9 dollars. I made a detailed medication chart, removed scatter rugs, and prayed to God that all would go well.

We asked many questions about the discharge plan, and called the surgeon's office more than once with any questions we had. You see, I am a nurse, but Steve has never been through such an invasive surgery as this, and what did I know? We wanted to be knowledgeable and prepared.

Two weeks after the surgery, we went for our post-op visit. I had two areas of concern on the discharge plan that I thought would help the next person. I saw the office manager to make that suggestion.

This is what advocacy is all about.

How can we be better advocates without feeling like a burden?

1. Before going to your HCP, make a list of questions you have, no matter how small

2. Get a second opinion when you want to be sure about a serious health issue
3. Take notes and bring a note book that has all your medical information in it, or update
4. Think simple, remember the "squirrels are in the woods, not the zebras." Use Google to look up information but keep it in perspective and look at reputable sites like Mayo Clinic.
5. Remember, you are important and so is the person you are caring for.

Another area that warrants your attention for self-advocacy is setting up an on-line portal for your medical information. I have downloaded the app from my Medicare advantage plan and have entered medications, allergies, and doctors.

Unfortunately, the doctors you see may not all be under one organization. My Chart by Epic allows me to digitally schedule lab tests, radiology, and specialist visits all under one app. I am able to combine other health care organizations on this app.

I still love paper, so I have a small notebook where I keep dates of new diagnoses, and when medications are started. This form of organization allows you to give an accurate account of your medical concerns so your health care provider can manage your care.

What is a Nurse Practitioner?

Nurse practitioners (NP) have become a household word and they have been at the forefront of providing medical care in all areas of health care. We are, first, a registered nurse with a bachelor's degree in Nursing from a 4-year accredited school. We then went on and completed advanced academic and clinical experience at the master's level (3-5year training) and is licensed by the State Board of Nursing. Our practice emphasizes health promotion and maintenance, disease prevention, counseling, and patient education.

As health care providers, NPs are trained and qualified to:

- Obtain health histories and perform physical exams
- Diagnose and treat common illnesses and injuries
- Recognize complicated medical conditions that require referral to specialists
- Manage chronic medical conditions such as diabetes, and hypertension
- Order and interpret diagnostic tests, including lab tests and X-rays
- Prescribe medications and other treatments
- Advise on how to prevent disease
- Offer education and counseling to assist in lifestyle changes
- Give vaccinations
- Refer to community resources and agencies

An NP can own and run clinics, be an attending clinician for hospice patients, and hold many different specialties from Acute Care to Pediatrics. NPs are also getting further degrees in a Doctor of Nursing (DNP). With the aging of the Baby Boomers and the shortage of physicians, the DNP is becoming the focus of medical care. This program is designed to produce leaders in Nursing. The role does not make an NP a "doctor," but the NP possesses the highest level of nursing expertise so that she/he can work either in a clinical or academic setting; or a leadership role upon obtaining the required credentials. They play an essential role in producing innovative programs that are economically sound. They learn to use evidence-based medicine in practice as well as in technology.

I have learned throughout the 40 years while working in home care, that caregivers were not well-informed of how to take care of many medical conditions that they could confront in the frail older adult or disabled. I found aides, nurses, and caregivers asking the same questions, and I dealt with teaching the same information over and over; thus, the impetus for me to write this book! I thought it was also important for me to help more than one person at a time and to write this "how to" book was the way to do it.

Ben Franklin has been quoted as saying "an ounce of prevention, is worth a pound of cure." By making this information available for all caregivers, then I have done my job as a clinician. This book can also help healthcare providers all over the world who are dealing with the disabled and older adult by reducing the number of patients calls they receive throughout the day for common problems.

Life happens so fast, and if you blink, you will miss it! And here we are, at the time we need to take care of us as we are aging, or take care of a friend, a family member or a child.

When the caregiver takes on the care of the older adult or disabled person, it's almost like bringing a new old baby into the home, but they don't come with instructions!

So, sit back and let me show you some practical applications you can use when caring for someone who is disabled, be it your mom, dad, sister, child, friend or yourself. I would recommend reading the entire book when you first get it. Little tidbits that you have read will help you know what to do along the path of caring and will help prevent medical crises.

To join my community, you can find Nancy the NP on google and social media. Please subscribe to my YouTube channel, "Caregiver Success" for instructional and inspirational videos. You can download teaching tools on my Facebook page: Facebook.com/CaregiverSuccess. Watch for the audio book coming out in the near future.

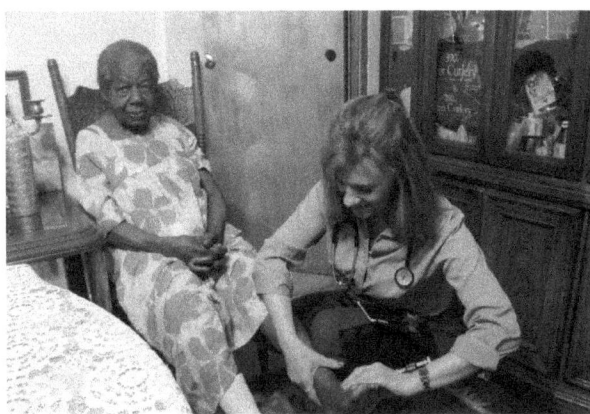
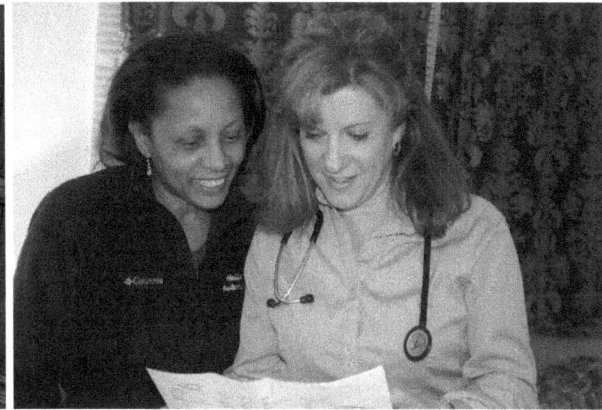

Background:

When I was a home care nurse for over 20 years, I wondered how a clinician could order medicine for a rash or treat a medical problem he/she has not seen. This problem was the impetus that led me to get a nurse practitioner certification and a master's degree in Nursing back in 1999. I realized that if caregivers were taught what to do to prevent problems, they could eliminate unnecessary suffering, medications, and ER visits. Also, I could treat the patient by seeing what the problem was by actually visiting the person in their homes.

After a few positions working as a nurse practitioner in primary care, I decided it was time to start a house calls company, called "Mobile Family Health Nurse Practitioner Care, PLLC in May 2010, and become the clinician who was treating that rash. I formed a medical referral network consisting of services for my patients: lab, ultrasound including echocardiogram, doppler testing, EKG, x-ray, dentistry, podiatry, optometry, aide referrals, rehabilitation, social work, hearing evaluations and behavioral health.

I took care of the young adult through age 106. I worked as the medical attending for my patients through the United Hospice of Rockland, signing death certificates for my patients. From this experience, I gained many practical nursing applications beyond what I learned in nursing school. It is time to share all these teachings to help you succeed as a caregiver.

My company merged with Vytalize Health in 2017 where I was the VP of Operations, and work with clinicians and their staff integrating wellness programs for Medicare patients and providing chronic care management and behavioral health programs.

The medical arena has changed where less hospitalization is the gold standard for Medicare. Hospitals are getting penalized if patients return to the facility within 30 days of discharge. Going to the hospital also leads to other medical problems such as exposure to other diseases. The idea is to avoid a medical crisis by thinking ahead so your loved one can remain home and be cared for there.

So, let's get started!

How to use this book:

The first section is full of tips and tools I have organized for you- It's all here for you to use as a caregiver; from how to make a bed with someone in it, to devices, like a magic sheet, that could make your life so much easier with positioning in bed.

The second section is about medical conditions that can occur in the older adult. This information is to be used in partnership with your healthcare provider (HCP) to help solve medical problems.

Section I

TIPS AND TOOLS TO CARE FOR THE OLDER ADULT/DISABLED

Who are We Caring for?
Why Should We Look our Best?

Ms. G met me at the door for a home visit. She is 86 years old and due to multiple medical problems; she does not drive; but she manages to "put her face on" every day- no matter how she feels. She has a box of cloth flowers to match every outfit. She dyes her hair red, puts on her blue eye makeup and wears cool, dangling earrings. She found that the one thing she can still do well is to teach Sunday school to second graders.

The pictures below are in the living room of my patient's home. There are pictures of her laughing with her children, her husband in an army uniform, and visions of many happy times in her life. Although she now suffers from dementia, she still enjoys when her daughters who come to dye her hair and bring her new lipstick. The daughters said their mom always liked to look her best. They keep her engaged by having her comb her own hair and apply her lipstick. A most important part of daily care for women is to remove unwanted hair from their face; so, make sure there are no stray gray hairs!

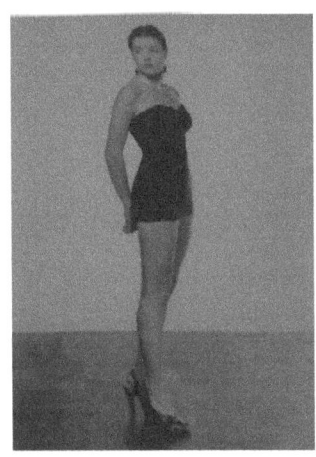 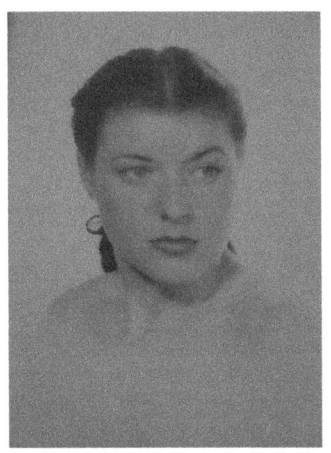 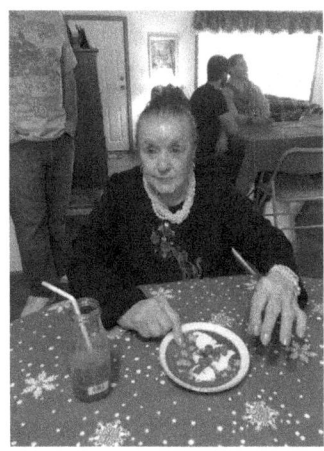

It is important for the person to "feel good" about how they look and that they feel they can maintain old habits. It helps to let them perform any form of activities of daily living, such as washing their extremities or applying body lotion to maintain movement of arms and fingers. If Dad liked to wear a bow tie, then let **him** clip it on!

Finding Your Purpose as an Older Adult

Finding your purpose at any age is important. Our purpose changes throughout our lives. First, I was a daughter, then a wife, a mother, a nurse practitioner, educator, business owner, nana and now author! We all have something to contribute, especially as we get older and wiser.

One of my patients loved to paint and design, so she started painting canes that she sold. Some were leopard print; others were of flowers, or stripes- any design to match an outfit. Other services our seniors can do is to knit hats for the homeless or the local hospital or bake for church functions. I had one patient, Ms. K., at 94, who was so astute with interpreting bills from her medical insurance, that she started helping her friends understand them and know whether they were correct.

I know a 94-year-old woman who is working in a Food Mart in the independent living facility where she lives. Her son says she is so sharp and engaged during the day because she has found her purpose. She has a reason to get up in the morning and the residents count on her to be there.

It is a good idea to have a chalkboard on the wall- where you can write the Day, Month and Year and change it daily. Make sure to bring up this information throughout the day by pointing to the board, to set reminders and reinforcement. A calendar that has a magic board (found in most craft stores) is good to write tasks and reminders for the present day.

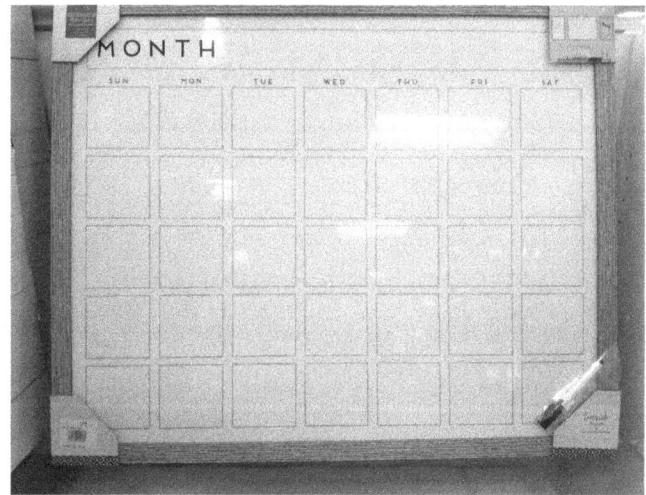

Having a "Bio Board" on the wall near where the person resides is good for all the aides to see. It goes something like this: "Meet Martha Smith- she was born during the depression in 1929, helped her parents raise her 7 brothers and sisters as the oldest…. she was the only one in her family to go to college and was the first female chemist. She loved to cook, travel and knit. She loves Frank Sinatra and old movie classics." The board can also show Ms. Smith's accomplishments, awards, degrees, etc.

This board allows all who meet her, to see who she was and what she likes. It allows the portrayal of the person as a contributing, living being even as she lies in the hospital bed, confused and disengaged.

Playing music that reminds the person of their past, or showing old pictures from an album can jog some memories. Maybe the person loved to paint, play piano, sing, draw, knit, etc. Try to tap into these innate thoughts to stimulate memory. I have found coloring books in craft stores that are cheap and fun. The books may help with engaging the person and lead to some conversation.

A poor personal connection is when an aide has very little verbal contact with a person with dementia. Sometimes it is because of a language barrier. It is much more beneficial for this person to have an aide that speaks the same language and is interactive so that he/she feels connected.

Taking Care of the Caregiver

Before we talk about the patient, let's talk about you, the caregiver. It takes patience, acceptance, unselfishness and time to take care of someone else when you have a life full of commitments of your own. I cannot emphasize enough that you need to take time for yourself for several reasons. People under excessive stress, develop their own set of medical problems. I have seen the caregiver "crash and burn" before the patient does. The caregiver becomes ill if elderly himself and sometimes dies before the patient does.

Think of it like being on an airplane and the airline stewardess is showing you how to apply the oxygen mask to yourself. Notice that if a child is sitting next to you, the stewardess says to put the mask on YOU first, then on the child. The same scenario goes for the caregiver. If you do not "put the oxygen mask on you first" before the person you are caring for, you will have a little reserve to get up and do it all again the next day causing caregiving to be ineffective.

It is not easy being the 24/7 person someone depends on. Even if an aide is living with your loved one, any problems, day or night become a concern for the family member. Sometimes, it is only one family member who is taking care of the person even when there are many that could help or be available. The daughter or son also has her/his own family responsibilities and may have a full-time job as well. I had a daughter who emailed us almost every day from Florida about her mom who is living in New York with a 24-hour aide.

There are a few ways of keeping your own preservation as a caregiver. Maintaining old friends and relationships is key; even if once a month, plans are in place to socialize. I was the HCP for the husbands of 4 women. They met at an Alzheimer's Association meeting where they gathered weekly on

Mondays for one hour. There, they got the support and tools they needed. Over the years, they remained friends even after their spouses had passed.

It is also important to have medical checkups regularly and maintain a healthy living by eating right and getting rest. Networking in the community for support can help you feel connected and feel like you are not alone. Take a little time for yourself.

Self-care can come in many forms. We all need to do self-care of some kind every day! As a senior myself, I have a benefit program for exercise called "Silver Sneakers." It is a FREE program that encourages movement.

I use prayer as my daily morning ritual. Sometimes I listen to spiritually-based podcasts like, Walking with Purpose (www.walkingwith purpose.com). Walking with Purpose is a virtual or in-person Bible study for adult women, young adult women and girls. The website states "Our Bible studies provide relevant content that takes timeless truths from Scripture and applies them to daily life." The Spotify app provides "WWP" podcasts you can listen to while you multi-task.

I enjoy baking, lighting a candle, listening to music, diffusing lavender essential oils, singing, dancing, gardening and creating art from nature. I love to find periods of self-joy like these.

One thing that is certain is that if we all live long enough, we are going to have some medical problems. By having yearly physicals, dental care, eye exams, and vaccinations, etc., we can catch something that is treatable before it causes permanent disease. As a caregiver, the person you are caring for hopes to have you around for them.

Try to take time to get out to your place of worship, join an art class or go for a daily walk. Work out time with other family members to come by so that you can get out for a set time, that you can count on. Respite for the caregiver will give strength and a positive outlook. It also keeps your identity- who you were BEFORE you were a caregiver.

When a loved one gets sick, it is good to hold a family meeting with siblings, a parent, etc. If possible, everyone should take part in the care of the person. I have seen families split up duties such as taking care of the finances, who gives the bath, who manages the medications; and even moving the person from home to home for a 3-month period to give other caregivers respite. It is difficult to be the sole caregiver with no one to bounce ideas and problems off of.

Other Matters to Help the Caregiver

(How to help get a good night's sleep)

Make your bedroom an "oasis of peace and rest." Your bed should be for sleep and sex. If there is laundry, a computer and bills around, remove them from your bedroom. When retiring to bed, it is not a good time to watch the news and other matters that bring on worry and stress. Having a good night's sleep can reduce your weight, your blood pressure, prevent diabetes and improve your overall well-being. The National Sleep Foundation recommends between 7 and 9 hours of sleep every night.

- start to wind down 15 minutes before you go to bed. Tuck Dad in, finish a few chores and relax by yourself for a few minutes
- get a fan or download an app from your phone for "white noise"- like ocean sounds
- If you must have your cell phone nearby, put it across the room, so you prevent getting exposed to its blue light
- get a comfortable pillow
- consider earplugs or eye mask
- keep a monitor near your bed, if need be, so you can hear Dad in the other room

- wear sweat wick PJ's
- have blinds or dark curtains to keep out the light
- try to go to bed at the same time every night
- if you have a pet, put a shirt that smells like you on the floor, so he sleeps there
- put a pen and paper near your bed for quick writing of thoughts buzzing through your head
- Avoid caffeine or alcohol a few hours before sleep as it may keep you awake, as well as any fluids
- If you suffer from chronic sleep problems, consider melatonin 3-5 mg or L-tryptophan, or see your HCP for medical help.

The Family Leave Act (FMLA) allows a family member to take off time from work, when needed, in order to care for their family member or if they are ill or need more care. I have completed the FMLA forms for many families. This form is obtained from the Health Resources Department at your employment. It is a form that indicates who is the person that needs the care, and what the medical problems are that requires you to leave work for a period of time to take care of him/her. By filling out the FMLA, it is a legal document that prevents the risk of losing your job. It needs to be completed by your HCP and kept on file by your HR Department. It is a good idea to keep a copy for yourself.

Ways to Increase Activity for the Caregiver

In order to prevent injury, it is important to keep the body in shape and joints limber. One thing that I cannot emphasize enough is how important it is to stretch every day. When I get out of bed, if I do not stretch for at least 5 minutes, I feel stiff all day. I also have more of a tendency to pull a muscle somewhere. Stretching increases range of motion, reduces stress and reduces the risk of injury. You do not need any equipment, and you can do it wherever and whenever you want.

Get yourself a Yoga mat and put on comfortable clothes. Make sure to include 2 to 3 stretches for each muscle group: back and shoulders, head and neck, arms, legs, and feet. Hold your stretches for at least 15 to 30 seconds and do not bounce. Stretching should be part of your routine, and it should not be painful. If something hurts, cut back on that exercise to prevent injury (see the following pages).

Meditation and learning to be in the present are great ways to perform self-care. (Check out my video: "JUST BREATHE" on my YouTube channel, Caregiver Success.)

ANN (NANCY) RHODES, APRN-BC

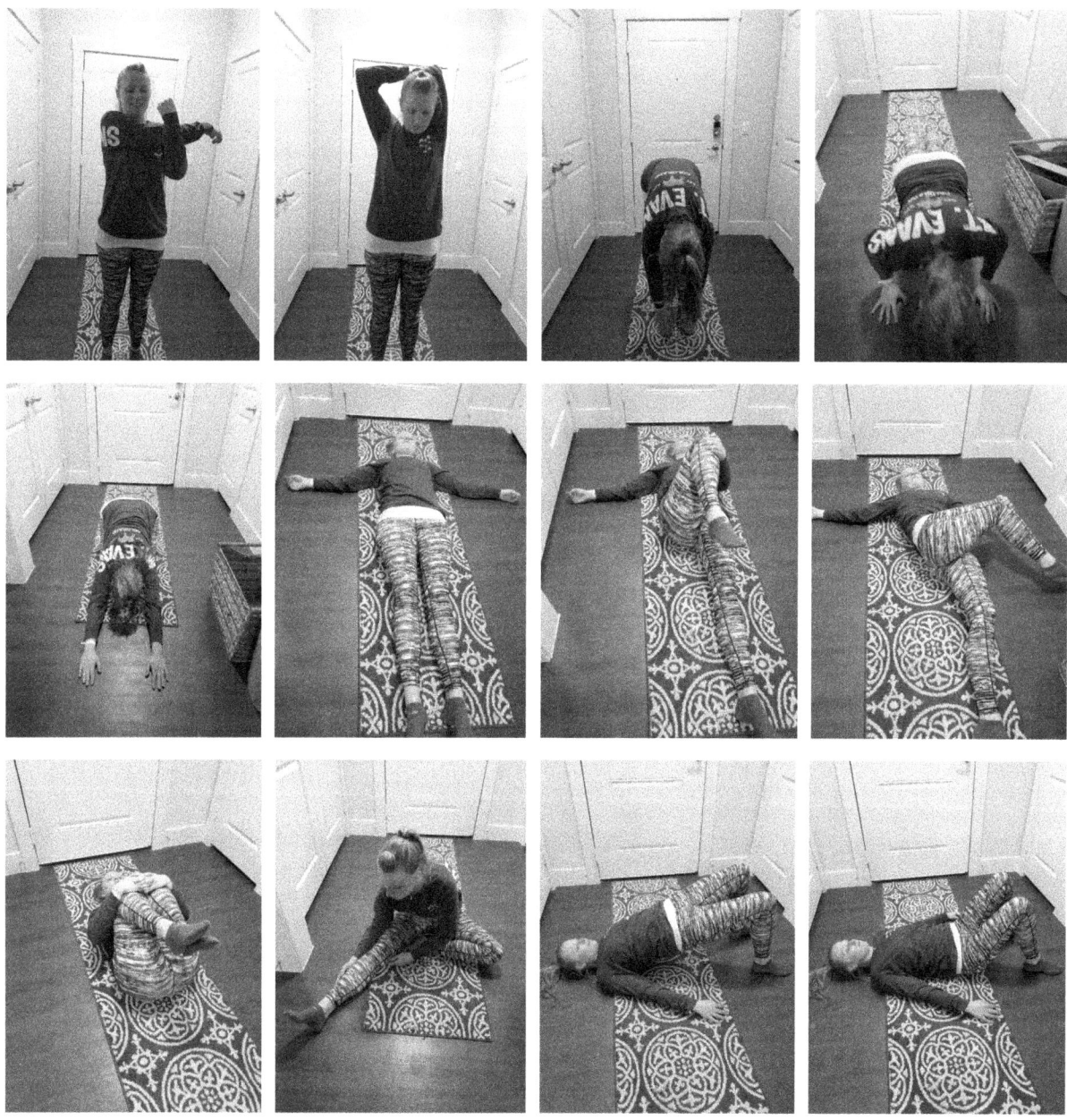

(If it is difficult getting down on the floor, do these exercises lying on a bed; be sure to repeat exercises on right and left sides)

Cardio and Endurance Training

What better way to lower your blood pressure, get more energy and stamina, and reduce stress but with cardio. This type of exercise increases your heart rate for a period of time. It is recommended to do moderate intensity (brisk walking) most days of the week. If you are the primary caregiver for Mom, have someone watch her for 30 minutes while you walk around the neighborhood or nearby park. It will get your head on straight before the day starts and make your outlook positive and productive.

Strength Training

Ok, we are not talking about becoming "Arnold." What this exercise does is helps build lean muscle which makes you stronger. Put a basket of 5-8-10 and 12 lb. weights and some bands near the TV. After Mom has turned in, take a few minutes to watch a funny show and lift some weights. If you do not have or cannot afford weights, consider lifting heavy books or a few cans of vegetables. Take an old gallon milk container and fill it with water sealing the lid with glue- now you have a real weight that costs you nothing to buy!

Random acts of exercise should be part of your day:

- Keep an extra pair of sneakers in the car. When going shopping, park further away from the store allowing you to walk a longer distance. If you have time after loading up the car, take a 10-minute walk around the parking lot.
- While talking on the phone, you can be walking around the house.
- To burn 150 calories, it takes 20 minutes of running, or shoveling snow; 35 minutes of raking leaves or a 2-mile walk. If you cannot walk outside, get creative and turn on some music, and dance!

Get Connected

In our community, we have a professional aging network where professionals who work with the elderly gather to network and share their contacts. The meetings are held monthly in various facilities across the county, such as nursing homes. The room is packed with elder lawyers, administrators from nursing homes, home health agencies, clinicians, etc.

For the caregiver, the Office of the Aging in your county is a good place to start finding connections. This office knows of home health agencies, mental health clinics, house calls programs, Medicaid office, social workers, office for the visually impaired, etc. With these connections, the caregiver will find more networks to help her/him be a successful caregiver.

If your parent has Alzheimer's Disease, you can google "Alzheimer's Association" and find your local chapter. Do not forget to consider your local church or synagogue for community support and volunteers. Another service available would be the Veteran's Association if your parent was a veteran. Medication could be completely covered; and you could have a nurse practitioner visit the home under this program.

A home health agency is a certified organization that provides visiting nurses, social workers, physical therapy, occupational therapy, and speech therapy. If your parent was recently in the hospital, they would be qualified for these services that last a few months or longer depending on their medical condition and progress. They can provide an aide paid for by Medicare Part B for a few hours a day, but for a short duration.

A recent hospitalization for pneumonia or a knee replacement, for example, is a medical reason for those services to come to the home. The person does need to be homebound, meaning it is taxing and difficult to get out to medical care. Home care services can continue indefinitely if there is a nursing skill such as the care for a monthly urinary catheter change.

Learn About Your Community

It is really important when Mom has either moved closer to you or you to her community, that you learn about the resources around you. If you are looking for a house calls company to come to the home, a good locator is American Academy of Home Care Medicine. Once you google this, you will be asked put in the zip code for your area. Hopefully, there is a clinician that can come to your home. Word of Mouth never fails- reach out to friends with similar situations with parents. Once the word gets out that someone is making house calls, it spreads like wildfire.

Let's talk more about the Alzheimer's Association. Over the years, my company took care of many patients with dementia and Alzheimer's Disease. Through our local chapter, they have multiple support groups for the caregiver and for those in early through late stages of the disease. The groups are led by a social worker who helps members speak about their concerns and problems. The support group in Rockland County of which I attended, was full of caregivers who were looking for solutions to some of their present problems. What I loved about the group was that everyone shared ideas and programs to help each other.

Get Organized

When your parents move into your home, it is a good idea to get organized. Rolling Tupperware stackable containers that act like drawers keep things organized and visible. You can organize items for bathing, wound care, incontinence pads, bed linens, etc. If possible, remove carpeting in the bedroom to keep the environment germ-free. Remove scatter (loose) rugs. Arrange pictures of past events for the person to be able to view. Consider getting a semi-electric bed or a commode, if appropriate.

(Check information section of "Fall prevention - inside" for more changes to the home).

Keep all your equipment receipts and user manuals together in a box or folder. Depending if your mother is on oxygen or other equipment, you will need the proper cleaning tools based on manufacturer instructions. Keep the daily log book close by for easy recording. Does your mother have a cell phone or Lifeline set up, so she can call for help?

Consider taking a CPR (Cardiopulmonary Resuscitation) class for basic life support/choking prevention. You can find this training at your local ambulance corporation or college. If you have taken the course before, there is a refresher online at a low cost.

Some tips for an emergency:

If your mother has a DNR, place it visibly on the refrigerator so the paramedics can find it easily.

If you are having an aide taking care of your mom, make a list of all contact numbers for family members she should call in case of an emergency.

Consider getting a medic alert bracelet, so if she goes out and there is an emergency where 911 is called, they will have some contact information on the bracelet. File of Life is a medical card you can buy online and have on the refrigerator. It contains all the medical information the first responder would need about the person. This information could save time and save a life.

Create an instruction sheet for the aide in case of an emergency:

- If the person is not responding, first call 911, THEN the family (calling 911 first is the right thing to do). The paramedics will quickly decide if it was an emergency. If the person is unresponsive and she has a DNR, make sure the aide knows to show it to them. If the DNR is not present and your mother needs CPR, they will begin CPR immediately.
- The aide is to call their agency next
- If there is a fire, make sure she knows where the fire extinguisher is and how to use it: review the technique called: P-A-S-S on YouTube
- If the fire is in another room, close the door of that room and place a wet towel at the bottom of the door
- If the person can walk, take her out of the home as quickly and calmly as you can
- If the person cannot walk, and she is in a hospital bed, crank the bed to the lowest level. If someone is in the home to help, remove the sheets from the bed, and gently lower her to the floor with the sheets.
- Pull her down the hall and /or down the steps carefully to get out of the building.
- If the aide can call for help, she may get assistance from someone, if in an apartment building.

In some counties in the USA, they have a registry for the first responders to quickly obtain important information (which is kept confidential) about those who live independently with limited mobility. By registering online, these individuals are connected with their local emergency personnel who will formulate a response plan in case of major weather or disaster in the community where they live. Just call your local Office of the Aging, or check out the National Council on Aging.

Items to have in the home when the person moves in:

Temporal or oral thermometer
Steri-strips
Saline wound wash
Large cotton men's socks
Disposable vinyl gloves
Band-Aids - all sizes
Non-stick dressings
Body lotion: unscented
Corn starch
Robitussin sugar-free (with no letters on the bottle)
Local Office of the Aging Services Book
Wet wipes (such as Prevail Adult washcloths)
Spiral notebook for daily patient log information
A fire extinguisher that is updated
A Log Book

This is a good time to talk about keeping track of daily activities.
I have found, as a clinician, that when visiting the home, it is a lot easier if there are daily records of a few things:

- What did the person eat today?
- How was her sleep last night?
- Did she have a bowel movement today, and if not, when and how much

- How much fluid did she drink?
- How is her skin?
- Did she take her medications?
- Did she have any change in her usual day, like congestion, vomiting, new pain, crying?

By keeping this log, when staff changes, it allows daily communication between them and the family. It could be a three-ring binder with pages or a notebook. You can make columns with check spaces or can be free form writing. This method is harder to follow, however based on the person's handle on the English language and penmanship.

I found this great spiral bound book called "The Patient's Checklist," written by Elizabeth Bailey, the patient advocate for preparation related to going to the hospital. She used the concept of checklists with tabs on the side of the book for easy find: "before you go, what to bring, medication list, insurance, family and doctor contacts, etc.

GroupMe is an app you can download onto your phone. It is a program that allows all family members near or far, to communicate about the person on a daily basis by going onto their own private application. They can discuss what she ate that day, how she is doing in the hospital, and the like. It is password-protected, so only people given permission is allowed to get onto the site.

In addition, your HCP probably has an online account where all your medical information, including lab, radiology tests, vaccinations, medications, doctor affiliates, etc. are all in one place. A broader phone app platform is MyFHR., where you can connect all the providers, even once that are not in the same network.

Your Aide

When you hire an aide from a local agency, she/he could be from any country. Some of them work in America for years without returning home to their families. Nellie, for instance, took care of one of my patients for 5 years. Ms. S., the patient, did not speak, was up most of the night due to insomnia and agitation; and needed undergarments changed every 3 hours. Nellie was from Ukraine, about 60 years old.

She had a home of which she showed me pictures. Her two children, in their 20s lived there and were responsible for the care of the home and the bills. Nellie would FaceTime her children weekly to keep in touch about family issues there. She had not seen them for over 5 years, only to go home after the patient passed away.

The patient's daughter would visit on Sundays, so Nellie had a day off to go to Brooklyn to see some aide friends she had made while Skyping. It was a very isolating time for her as she had no one to talk with most of the time. She managed to take some courses online and lost about 50 lb. She was a great cook and had adapted meals from solids to soups and puréed as Ms. S's condition changed. I would visit once a month to see Ms. S. and would spend time with Nellie- having a meal with her just for the company. She appreciated this as the years went by.

I have found, the more the aide is made part of the family, the commitment and trust can become very strong. We have become very aware of cultural diversity and how to accept people from all places. It is, at times, harder for the older generation to accept people of all colors, I have noticed. With the language barrier and cultural differences, I have seen all types of responses by patients about their aides. Some love them, and some wished they could be alone without any help.

I make sure to compliment the aide on the care she is giving and does give suggestions if I do not agree with how some things are done. I will leave written instructions, so if there are different aides, they can share the information with each other.

An important point that needs to be made is that the person being cared for needs to be respected. Just because the person is old and frail, cannot speak and may be incontinent, does not mean the person can be called "honey" or sweetie." It is common for caregivers to use these names instead of the patient's proper name, such as Mr. Smith. If the person says, "please call me John" then it is important to use his name when addressing him.

Finding an Aide/ Companion- Private

You may need to get an aide to help in the home for a period of time. Medicare can provide some hours of care if there is a skill in the home such as a visiting nurse or therapist. It may be time to consider someone there for more hours, and that requires shopping around to find out cost (as this is an out-of-pocket expense).

I had worked with companions that, when the patient was no longer walking, became incontinent, and needed total care, they were not trained to handle this type of change in the person. I had to alert the families that it was no longer safe for the patient if the companion is not qualified to care for him/her. The companion was cheaper as the patient did not have that many needs, but once the patient is up all night, needs the bed changed with the patient in it, or needs turning every 2 hours, for example, the cost of the aide increases. It is also important that the aide is able to get rest/ time off so as to not burn out. This is where 12-hour shifts may be needed.

Here are some questions you may want to ask the individual you are interviewing:

- How long have you been caring for people at home?
- When was the last time you worked in this capacity?
- May I have two references: name, address, phone number, of previous cases and why did you leave?
- Have you worked with very ill patients that are bedridden?
- Have you taken care of someone who is dying?
- How did that feel for you?
- Do you know how to take care of a bedbound person?

(see section in the beginning of the book – What does Compassion Mean?)

What is your knowledge of:

- Changing bed linens with the person in the bed
- Applying under pads
- Placing a person on a bedpan
- Changing undergarments/ adult incontinence products
- Assisting with the use of a urinal
- Applying a condom catheter
- Positioning a patient in bed
- Mouth care
- Skin care
- Complete bed bath
- Taking care of a Foley catheter, oxygen, nebulizer, etc.?
- Washing hair in bed
- Have you ever given a person medication?
- Have you ever given a suppository?

- Do you know how to safely transfer a person from bed to wheelchair / commode and back to bed?
- Do you smoke?
- Do you drive? Do you own your car?
- How do you feel about preparing meals? What type of foods do you know how to cook?
- What would you do if the person you were caring for fell?
- If they stopped breathing?
- If there was a fire in the house?
- How do you feel about being asked to provide care in the middle of the night?
- Explain the type of sleeping accommodations that you plan to provide for the aide. Are these acceptable to you?
- Do you mind animals? Dogs and cats? How much do you charge: per hour? day? month?

You may want to draft a written agreement, signed by all parties, indicating all responsibilities and the fee to be paid.

What is Cultural Diversity?

When looking for a companion for your parent, take into consideration whether there are any cultural differences he/she may have. It is unfortunate, but I have seen older patients not like their aide because she/he was black, spoke broken English and primary language was French Creole, or that they do not like their cooking because it is not "American cooking." I have also experienced the embracement by an Irish woman of her aide, who cooked Italian food for her, and she loved it. Many times, as time goes on, the person finds that the aide is lovely, kind and has become her friend; suddenly, the aide is now "just like her."

Cultural diversity is defined, according to Wikipedia, as "the quality of diverse or different cultures"; it also means "the variety of human societies or cultures in a specific region." America and many countries all over the world have become their own "melting pots." I have walked into a home seeing pots boiling on the stove, with all types of smells and seasonings. I have asked what they are cooking and can I have a taste, just to be a part of their culture.

I have worked with a great program for finding caregivers, called "Lean On We." What I like about the website is you actually see the picture of the caregiver and hear her/ him speak about why they want to be your caregiver. You get to explore their rates, recommendations, credentials, specialties and skills, working locations, whether they have a car, etc.

This agency also provides emergency fill-ins should your caregiver not be available. Hiring a caregiver is a tax write-off, and they work with a payroll company that helps you, the employer, pay the caregiver, your employee. They work with long-term care programs as well. They service metro NYC, CT, and NJ. Their website is www.LeanOnWe.com.

The Art of Listening

There is something to be said about listening and not speaking. My mom always said, "you have one mouth and two ears, so you are meant to listen." One thing I have learned over the years when caring for people, is they want to be heard. When I first meet a new patient, I make eye contact, shake his or her hand, and address them by their proper name. If the daughter says "mom does not hear well," I smile and pull my chair closer to her, and make sure she can see my face so she can observe my gestures and body language for better communication. A funny suggestion I always say is "if you wear glasses, put them on so you can hear me better."

Another very important part of new communication is to examine the patient's ears for wax. Most of the time, a homebound person has not had her ear canals examined, sometimes for years. This may be gross to you, but I have removed rock-like two-inch long wads of wax that must have been in the ears for years! It is an extra task to remove the wax but is SO needed for good communication (and Medicare pays the clinician to remove it to boot!)

Once we have the proper introduction, I begin to ask pertinent questions to the patient about her home situation, like "how has everything been for you, and are you having any problems you would like to talk about today?" If a family member is present, as a husband, I can easily see how their relationship is by how they talk to one another; and also, by watching their body language. Rolling of the eyes, whispering behind his wife's head to me about something or just the fact of the family member leaving the room during intake, says a lot.

I continue to "peel the onion," beit the patient or the caregiver. By peeling the person layer, by layer, meaning, by seeing their mental, emotional, personal and physical status, I can determine what they may need and how I can help them. This does not happen at first glance, but evolves over time, with more home visits and after speaking to other clinicians, aides, family members, and the like.

I also observe the appearance of the caregiver. I noticed when visiting one of our patients who is 50 years old, and requires total care, by his wife, Susan, that she had gained quite a bit of weight, is no longer touching up her grays and her clothes looked disheveled. I would then ask how she was doing, is she getting any respite, and does she need help with anything.

As a result of my observation, I found out she is tired because her husband, Mark, needs range-of-motion exercises of his joints at least once daily and she cannot find anyone to help her, so she is doing it herself. Not only is she taking care of her two teenage kids after school, but she also cleans the home, she cooks meals, pays the bills, etc.

I immediately hit my network list and found a man who would love to help her out. I called Larry during the visit and had him speak with her so they could meet through me. Larry called me later and said he was going to the home almost daily to help Mark with these exercises. I realize this help was not everything Susan could use, but at least I saw something I could do to help her.

Sometimes, just touch is all someone needs. I always touch the person's arm and say a few words, like "see you soon" or "take care," to the person who is unresponsive in bed before I leave. Compassion is not something we give but what we get from others. I find that what I do and say to my patients is part of who I am and has given me a purpose in this life as a helper and problem solver.

Having no judgment when someone is a hoarder or lives in squalor allows me to focus on what is in front of me- the person. When a patient is confused and almost funny, it is important not to belittle them by laughing. I have told family members not to make fun or put down their family member, but to show respect and patience; remember who they were and who they are now.

When one of my patients would pass away, the family got a handwritten card thanking them for letting me care for their loved one, some of my memories of the person, and that I wish them peace. This gesture also helps us with closure as we say goodbye to another patient. I truly believe we get something from all the people who touch us as we touch them.

Advanced Care Planning

When the person became our patient, we would have a discussion about advanced directives, health care proxy and Do Not Resuscitate (DNR). If the person is capable of understanding the discussion, we ask her/him what their wishes are- if she were to stop breathing right here and now, would she want to be brought back to life by CPR.

Getting resuscitated does not bring the person back without complication. There can be broken ribs, a lacerated liver, a need for a ventilator to assist with breathing; and she may not regain consciousness. Depending on what state your parent lives in, a nurse practitioner may be able to sign the DNR. This document is to be placed on a refrigerator, so if 911 is called, the paramedics will know to look there so that the person's wishes are granted not to be resuscitated.

You can look online for the forms to complete a health care proxy for your state. This form is legal and binding as long as the two witnesses are over the age of 18 and neither one of them is the proxy. The person can fill in the blanks and check the boxes as to her wishes, as long as she is capable of understanding.

You do not have to be an older adult to have a health care proxy. Everyone should have one over the age of 18. It takes the burden off the spouse or child since the wishes were clearly documented. When a Will for our possessions is done, a health care proxy is usually included in the legal documents. This proxy can be changed at any time if the person's health changes or their proxy dies before them.

(Google "Health Care Proxy Forms)

Ageism

When we feel that we are discriminated at because of our age, a term called ageism has emerged. It is a prejudice of people against older people. All "isms" are conjured up by people- sexism and racism are two such examples. It is the denial we carry in our minds about aging that makes us try ways to look younger, such as getting Botox injections or using expensive skin creams. Social media has been turning this around. It has been great to see the older, or overweight woman or man portrayed as a vibrant, attractive part of our society. We need to continue to come up with alternative and better views on getting old, as we are all going in that same direction.

The World Health Organization (WHO) is initiating a movement about changing the view on getting old, and being proactive as we age by us first being preventive. There are things we can do so we can age but age well. Some things we can do, for instance, to stretch every morning, stop smoking, lose that belly that can give you diabetes, learn new things, and find your purpose. If we feel better about getting older, then we will age better and have a better quality of life. Also, stop making fun of yourself as you age, like saying "that senior moment" when you misplaced your keys. I misplaced my keys when I was a teenager. Was I having a "senior moment" then?

The Annual Wellness Exam

Medicare pays for a yearly wellness exam for seniors over the age of 65 at no cost. This exam is not an annual physical exam and does not require the patient to get in a gown. The purpose of the "exam" is to look at the "well you" and your world. What I love about this exam is that it focuses on health promotion and disease prevention and detection to help beneficiaries stay well. Many Medicare Advantage plans are also covering it, so if you do not have traditional Medicare, call your health insurance carrier and find out if you are eligible to have this exam.

The exam starts with checking your height, weight, pain screening, oxygen level, temperature, pulse, respiratory rate, and blood pressure. It goes on to include a cognitive screen, preventive care history, tobacco use screening, alcohol misuse screening and counseling, fall history, and depression screening, assessment of home safety, such as smoke detectors, and assessment of home clutter. It is time to talk about advanced directives and your medical wishes. The questions include your present home situation- are you widowed, live alone, have social supports. Are you able to perform all activities of daily living- cooking, shopping, bathing, paying bills?

At the end of the exam, you will receive a Personalized Prevention Plan (PPP) which includes all your medical problems and the medical /personal interventions suggested by your HCP, a list of screenings recommended for your age group based on smoking and sexual activity status from the US Preventive Services Task Force (USPSTF). Every year, this plan is updated.

This includes screenings you may need, such as hypertension control, smoking cessation, (if you are a smoker), and a test to check for syphilis (if sexually active and had more than one partner recently). You will also receive recommendations for any vaccines due.

Referrals to programs such as physical therapy for fall prevention and support groups are also part of the program. Every community has some senior program directory through the Office of the Aging or county office.

In addition, you and your HCP can be part of Chronic Care Management (CCM) and Behavioral Health Integration (BHI) programs. CCM involves being over 65, and have 2 or more chronic medical problems that is at least one year old, such as hypertension and high cholesterol. The program is promoting a better quality of life and improved health, as well as lower costs for eligible patients.

Many Medicare Advantage plans have financial incentives when you do preventive programs, so take advantage of it, if it is available to you.

The beneficiary has access to the electronic medical records portal where your HCP records all of the medical tests and information, 24/7 on call to a service that provides a nurse practitioner to answer any questions after hours. There is some additional revenue for your HCP for behind-the-scenes integration of care: interpretation of your labs, speaking with other providers about your medical issues, writing letters on your behalf, FMLA forms, etc.

A Behavioral Health Integration Program involves a virtual team consisting of a nurse practitioner, social worker, and psychiatrist who discuss mental issues that are of concern for the patient and provide counseling, and medical treatment as necessary. The group discusses the treatment and progress on a monthly basis and as needed.

I found this service to be so important since many of my patients would not leave home due to mental issues such as depression and anxiety. We were able to improve their quality of life by bringing the program to them.

Medicare Part B also covers other preventive services:

- Bone mass measurements
- Cardiovascular disease screening
- Colorectal cancer screening
- Diabetes screening
- Diabetes self-management training
- Glaucoma screening
- Hepatitis C screening
- HIV screening
- Influenza, Pneumococcal, and Hepatitis B vaccines
- Intensive Behavioral therapy for cardiovascular disease
- Intensive Behavioral therapy for obesity
- Medical Nutrition Therapy
- Prostate cancer screening
- Screening for cervical cancer with HPV testing
- Screening for lung cancer with low dose computed tomography
- Screening mammography
- Screening Pap tests
- Screening pelvic examination (includes clinical breast exam)
- Ultrasound screening for Abdominal Aortic Aneurysm

So, ask your HCP about these screenings. You can visit CMS (Centers for Medicare and Medicaid Services) and search for Medicare Learning Network.

Burial and Funeral Plans- are you prepared?

Many of us do not give much thought to our burial plans. We plan for our children's college educations, vacations and our retirement but we do not plan for our own funeral and burial. Even our parents who we now may be caregivers for, may not have a plot or have set aside monies for a funeral. In addition, about 30% of the population has a will that states their wishes, and the other 70% does not. We also need to consider the various religious beliefs and their traditions, as they may be different than the Christian burial process.

It is not a subject many of us want to broach, but our immortality is inevitable. The reasons for not making these plans is fear and lack of education. Also, the wife wants to get things in order but the husband does not, so nothing happens. By not making plans, we have left the burden on those who are living and are dear to us. Now, our children have to make all the plans of do we bury or cremate? While they are grieving, they are in the throes of planning a funeral and burial.

Imagine that there were plans made and the bill was paid- your parents both agreed with cremation, picked out an urn and had purchased a plot and a funeral home. They had their music and readings in writing for their funeral service. It allows the children or family time to grieve because everything was planned and paid for.

An example of this was my in-laws. They purchased a cremation plan 10 years before they died. When my father-in-law died suddenly, all it took was a phone call to the company to collect the body, and in 2 weeks an urn arrived at our home. The same thing happened when my mother-in-law died in another state. A phone call was made and the body was collected, the urn appeared (the one she had picked out) two weeks later. They did have a burial plot so there was a service a few years later (the delay was because of the pandemic) and all 7 children and the extended family could attend without any disagreements.

Honestly, it was a wonderful experience. There are choices as to what one can do: in-ground burial, columbarium burial, a family estate (site for all generations) and a mausoleum burial.

In-ground Burial: requires a cemetery plot, a casket and a vault or urns for cremains as well as a memorial monument or marker.

Columbarium Burial- generally is an outdoor structure which provides niche spaces for urns with cremains. These are sealed behind marble slabs.

Family Estate – a custom designed burial plot that enables families to build lasting tributes for generations to come.

Mausoleum Burial- indoor or outdoor structure that provides a crypt (casket) space or a niche space for an urn with cremains. The crypt is sealed behind a marble "shutter front" slab and the niche can be sealed behind marble or glass.

It is important to make plans and to make them known to your loved ones. They will be happy you did.

BURIAL AND FUNERAL PLANS- ARE YOU PREPARED?

The average cost of a funeral and burial is **$8,300** up from $7,848, according to the latest data from the National Funeral Directors Association (NFDA). If you get a vault — required by many cemeteries — that number rises to $9,995. The average cost of a funeral and cremation is a little lower: **$6,280**.

What costs are involved with a funeral?

Depending on the type of funeral you choose, you may have to pay for a range of services and materials. The NFDA compiled the average price breakdown across the US, but you could pay more or less based on where you live.

Item	Cost	Description
Metal casket	$2,500	The average casket made from metal, fiberboard, fiberglass or plastic casket costs $2,500. But some mahogany, bronze and copper caskets can set you back as much as $10,000, according to the Federal Trade Commission.
Funeral service fee	$2,459	This fee covers the cost of the funeral home or cemetery's labor and equipment.
Vault	$1,695	The price of the protective enclosure the coffin rests in.
Cremation casket	$1,310*	The cost of the combustible container required for the cremation process.
Embalming	$845	The process of preserving a human body is often required for open-casket services or if the remains are set to be transferred interstate.
Funeral home staff	$550	An optional fee for enlisting the funeral home staff to assist with this service.
Facility usage	$475	If you want to use the funeral home's chapel for the viewing, you'll pay this fee.
Cremation fee	$400	The cost of cremating the body. Most funeral homes don't have crematoriums, so they need to outsource this to a third-party.
Hearse	$375	The charge for the vehicle used to transport the body from the funeral home to the cemetery.
Transportation	$395	The price of transferring the body to the funeral home or morgue.
Urn	$295	The price of the urn to hold the remains after they've been cremated.
Cosmetic preparations	$295	Funeral homes charge a fee for any cosmetic preparation relating to makeup application, clothing and hairstyling.
Memorial service extras	$195	The cost of printing pamphlets, prayer cards and other materials for the funeral.
Service vehicle	$125	The fee for transporting family members to and from the funeral.

(Go to the Glossary for "72 Decisions in 72 Hours")

The Bedridden Patient

How to make a bed with someone in it (an occupied bed):

First, gather:

- Disposable gloves
- A new set of bed sheets: fitted and top sheet
- Clean undergarment (if due for changing)
- New chuck (blue absorbent sheet)
- One sheet folded into a square to be used as a "draw" sheet

- Wash your hands
- Tell the person what you are going to do every step of the way, even if you are not sure she understands.
- If in a hospital bed, use the crank at the back of the bed and crank the bed up to your waist level. (be sure to bend your knees slightly and hinge your torso slightly forward so you don't hurt your back!)
- If the head of the bed is elevated, use the remote-control device to make the bed flat
- Put on a pair of disposable gloves
- Turn the person to the railing on the opposite side of you- and have her hold on, if able
- Put down the bed railing on your side
- Loosen the bottom sheet, and remove the top sheet
- If the person is soiled, this is the time to loosen the old undergarment and clean the right side of the patient using wipes or clean washcloth
- Pull the undergarment down

- Proceed to roll the soiled chuck, soiled undergarment, under sheets together and roll them under the person
- Now apply the new bottom sheet to the bed and add the draw sheet with chuck on top of it
- Roll those sheets together by first rolling them towards you but most of it you tuck under the person and soiled sheets
- If you can remove the soiled undergarment, this is the time to do it
- Be careful not to allow the soiled sheets to soil the new sheets
- Now have the person let go of the bed railing
- Put up the bed railing on your side of the bed
- Tell her to roll towards you
- This is when you roll the person over ALL the sheets until she can hold onto the rail you just pulled up
- Go to the other side of the bed
- Finish cleaning her on the left side now, and remove the soiled undergarments
- Remove the soiled sheets and chuck
- If everything was very soiled, you could apply a clean pair of gloves
- Proceed to pull the clean bottom sheet over, and roll out the new draw sheet and chuck with it
- Now fit the under sheet and smooth out any wrinkles in the sheets.

(Go to YouTube- "Caregiver Success" on "how to make a bed with someone in it")

How to position someone in bed:

- Remember always to tell the person what you are doing, even if he does not speak or understand
- If a person is bedridden, it is important, if he/she cannot move, to help him, using the support of joints, and keeping good body mechanics.

The areas of the body where the bone is close to the surface of the skin are called bony prominences. These areas are under the most pressure and at greatest risk for developing pressure sores. By positioning with wedges against the back and using pillows between the knees, and by turning the person every 2 hours from side-to-side, you can reduce the chance of causing skin breakdown.

- It is good to keep the person's head of the bed up 30 degrees, if possible.
- Also, use the knee gatch. By bending the knees, the person will not slide down the bed.

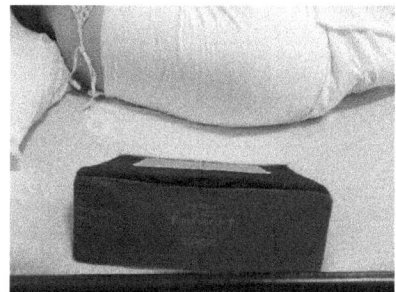
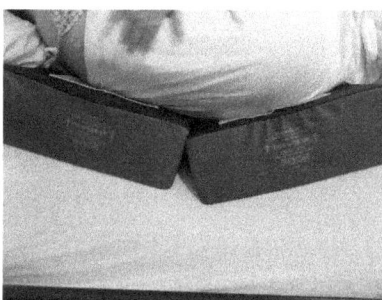
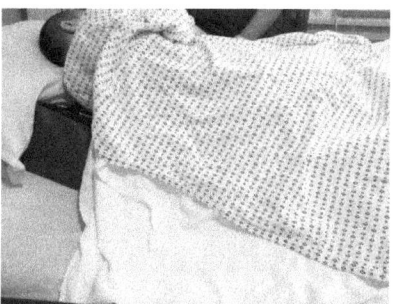
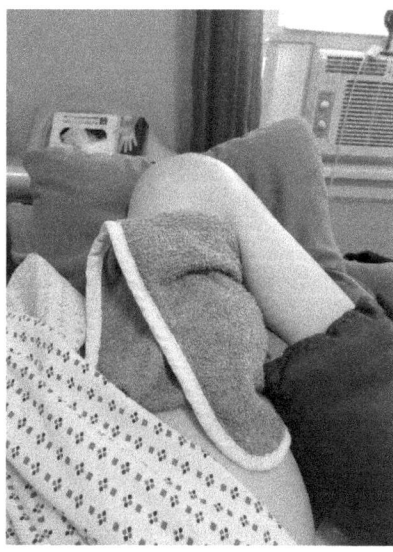

How to pull someone up in bed:

- A draw sheet is great for pulling someone up in bed
- Raise the bed to waist level for you using the crank at the bottom of the bed
- Make the bed flat using the remote
- If there is not a draw sheet under the person, place one there
- If you can get to the head of the bed, go there and tell the person to bend her knees to help you
- Grab both sides of the sheet under the patient at the head of the bed
- Gently but firmly pull the person up in bed until her head is almost to the top

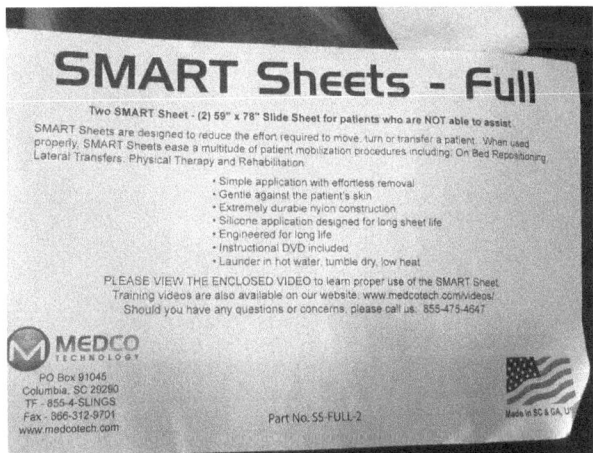 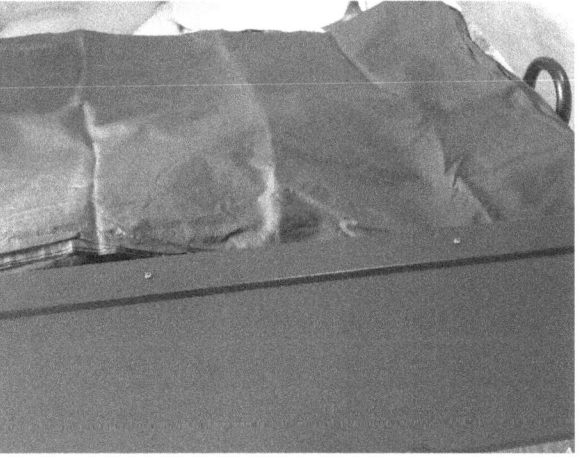

Smart sheets are designed to reduce the effort to move, turn or transfer a person. These sheets are slippery, so you can easily pull someone up in bed with one person and avoid any friction.

If there is someone to help:

- Have them go to the side of the bed opposite you and hold onto the draw sheet
- Prop a pillow up against the headboard to prevent hitting the head during transfer
- With person's knees bent, or not, on the count of 3, simultaneously both pull the person up in bed
- Raise the head and knee gatch after positioning the patient
- Ask the person if they are comfortable

How to change an undergarment in bed:

- If the person needs to be changed in bed, look under section: "changing bed with someone in it."
- It is best if the person can be transferred out of bed to a bedside commode, but if she can't:
- Put on disposable gloves
- Have the person stand for a second while you pull down the soiled undergarment
- Help them transfer to the bedside commode if needed
- If you are using pull-up undergarments, this is the time to put them on
- Once they are done on the commode, and if the person can stand, have them do so
- Use wipes to clean the penis first or the vaginal area, then move to the back; NEVER clean back to front
- Consider applying a barrier cream to the buttocks (like Desitine)
- Reapply the new garment (if there are straps on the side), then transfer back to bed
- Make sure to look at the skin for any redness or sores

Hair washing

Another important procedure and part of good hygiene is the washing of hair. It is not easy for an older person who is no longer able to get into a shower to have their hair washed.

There are products available such as dry shampoos. Shower caps with dry shampoo in them that can be applied to the head and left on for a period of time to help remove the oils from the hair. Nothing is better than good old shampoo and water.

How to wash someone's hair in bed:

This brings me back to a fond memory I have of an older nurse and mentor, Margaret Donne RN who worked with me in a home health agency for many years. She taught me how to use household items to wash hair in bed. You will need:

- Two large garbage bags
- Two large towels
- Plastic collecting device or bucket
- Large bowl with warm water
- Shampoo
- Vinyl gloves – one pair

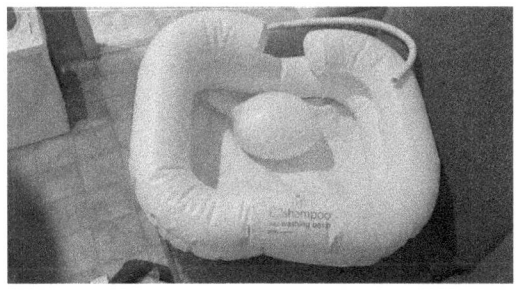

- Wash your hands
- Place the patient close to the edge of the bed where you will be setting everything up
- Insert two large rolled-up towels in a U shape with the U being sideways shaped like the letter "C"
- Now take those towels and gently place them in a large garbage bag
- Place the person's head on this garbage bag with the towels, so that the rolled towel is now under the neck and the other side of the towel goes around the head

- Place the bucket on the floor
- Drape another garbage bag, so it acts like a spout for the water to drain into the bucket
- Now you are ready to wash hair! Continue to wash and rinse until the hair and scalp are clean
- You can buy a device you can blow up, if you prefer, instead of the above method

(Go to YouTube, Caregiver Success- "How to wash someone's hair in bed")

How to give someone a bath in bed:

The idea is to wash one side of the body, placing towels on that side, in order to keep the bed dry and for drying off the extremities as you wash. This is a good time to inspect the skin for any new rashes or open areas. Put on some music, talk to the person and let them know what you will be doing and when. Do not forget to let them actively participate with the bath: brushing their own teeth, combing hair, using the washcloth.

You will need:

- Pair of vinyl gloves
- Washcloth and wipes
- Towel for the bed and towel for drying
- Pump soap
- A bowl of warm, clean water
- Body lotion- preferably without fragrance
- Corn starch

- Start with the face and go from "clean" to "dirty," leaving the private areas for cleaning for last

- Change the water a lot, as it gets soapy.
- Apply lotion to dry skin as you go
- If the person has skin folds in the abdomen and groin, put some cornstarch in the palms of your gloved hands, clap your hands together to remove some of the cornstarch, then gently pat the powdered gloved hand on the creases and folds. Cornstarch is great for keeping areas dry.

After the bath is a good time to change the linens and undergarments.
(See this process under "the bedridden patient." Section 1; also watch on my YouTube channel, Caregiver Success)

The bedridden patient requires special care since all care has to be done in bed. With the use of a Hoyer lift or a device called a transfer board, patients may be able to be taken out of bed to a chair, commode or shower chair.

How To Use a Hoyer Lift:

Do not be afraid to use a Hoyer lift alone. It is a great device for a person who cannot stand so that they can be transferred safely from bed to chair, and vice versa. In addition, it can reduce injuries to the caregiver.

Remember to talk to the person as you go through the process, even if they do not understand. Your calm voice and demeanor will make the experience less scary.

- Have the person in bed
- Have the wheelchair or chair you are transferring to, ready and nearby. If it is a wheelchair, put the brakes on
- Lower the bed rail
- Roll the Hoyer sling next to the person -head end toward the person's head
- Roll the person to the one side of the bed and push the sling up against a person's back

- Ask the person to hold onto the side rail near them
- Gently roll the person back over the sling and pull half of the sling through
- Gently roll the person back to be flat in bed; make sure the sling is positioned so the person 's head will be on the higher end of the sling
- Roll the Hoyer device with the wheels together under the bed
- Open the wheels on the base to stabilize the Hoyer lift
- Lock the wheels of the lift in place
- Using the metal lever near the middle of the lift, push it gently counterclockwise and slowly lower the sling apparatus down over the person until the apparatus is low enough to attach the loops
- Turn the metal lever clockwise to stop the device from lowering further
- Using the same-colored loops on all 4 sides of the sling, loop them onto the hooks on the Hoyer device
- Using the lever in front of you, begin to crank the Hoyer sling up. The person can hold onto the sides if she wants, or folds her arms in front of her
- Continue to crank the device up until the sling is suspending the person up enough for you to move the person away from the bed
- Now unlock the wheels of the Hoyer so it can move
- Pull the Hoyer device away from the bed with the person in the sling
- Keep the legs of the Hoyer apart for stability as you roll it to the chair
- Be sure to watch her legs that they do not hit the pole of the Hoyer in front of you
- Make sure the chair is either secured against a wall to prevent tipping, or if a wheelchair, make sure the wheels are locked
- Wheel the person to the chair and position the sling above the seat of the chair/ wheelchair
- Move the metal lever slowly counterclockwise and lower the person into the chair

- You may need another person to help adjust the sling before lowering the person into the chair, so she is upright. (You can go to the back of the chair and pull upwards on the sling if you are alone and can reach over the device to push the lever)
- Push the lever clockwise, once the person is in the chair to prevent the sling from lowering more
- Remove the sling loops from the device and pull away with the Hoyer lift
- The sling stays under the person until you want to transfer her back to bed
- You may need another person to help adjust the sling before lowering the person in the chair, so she is upright.
- Pull the lever to the left to close the wheel legs once you are done with the transfer
- Now the Hoyer can be stored until the return transfer

(Check out my YouTube video on using the Hoyer lift, on Caregiver Success)

The Hoyer I used in the video was an older model. It is important to feel safe with the transfer, and when possible, have someone assist you. Make sure you have the right size sling for the size of the person.

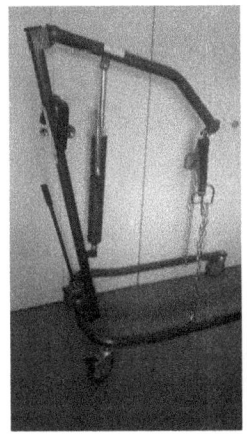
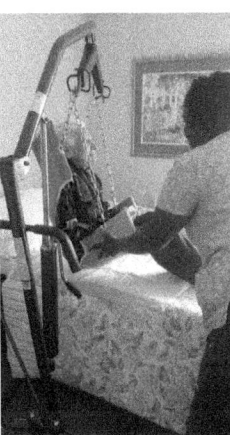
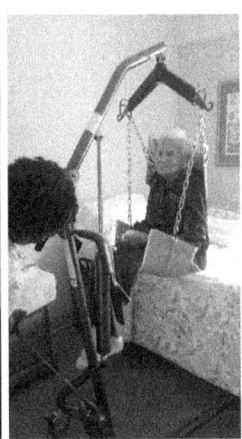
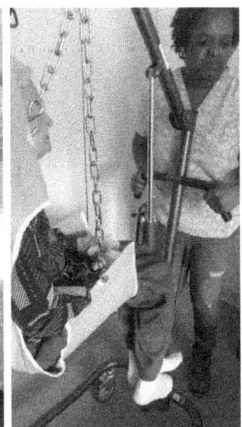
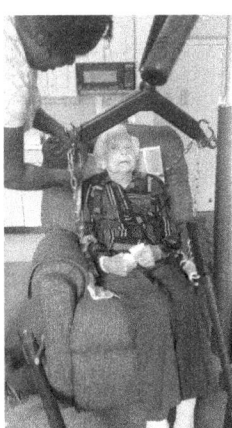

Stimulation for the bedridden patient:

When a person is bedridden, or goes from bed to chair, life can be pretty boring. Consider playing the person's favorite music during the bath, or have a diffuser of lavender on at night to help with sleep. Pictures should be everywhere, including the ceiling. You could have a large family picture of everyone waving- wouldn't that be great? Carve out some time from your busy day for mental stimulation time. This goes for children who cannot walk as well.

Change can be good

My Mother-in-law, Mary, had been living alone for over 2 years since her husband of 62 years passed away in 2017. She was always independent and was able to take care of all bills, writing checks and keeping up with her household in Florida. She agreed to have her oldest child, Donna, become her financial (Power of Attorney) POA so that when and if Mary could not carry out this function, it would not become a legal issue.

Last summer, Mary spent a month with us in Connecticut. She loved to cook. We have a large vegetable garden every year, and every year, we would make dilled pickles to zucchini bread. I can see us standing side by side chopping and chatting. She would drive (without a map) all over the tri-state area alone to visit her other 6 children.

Steve and I took his mom back to Florida in the fall. She would set up her Christmas tree, standing on a small ladder mentioning it was the last time she would do that as it was a hard project to do alone. We had been talking about moving all together and retiring to a warmer climate such as Delaware. Donna was going to move with us and be Mary's caretaker as time went on. She was adamant that she did not want to be a "burden" to any of us.

When the first addition of this book was released back in February 2020, we were all in a very different place. The COVID-19 Pandemic had been unraveling and causing the world to stand still. In August 2020, Mary was desperate to get up to Connecticut to live with us. No one knew what the future would bring. It was then, that I flew down on a 747 plane out of NY, one of 20 people on the plane, masked and aisles away from others, in order to get to Florida to drive her back to CT.

Over the next 8 days, we had a garage sale, fixed a dead car battery, had 2 doctors' appointments, packed up and cleaned the home, and had a party with her friends. We drove over 1200 miles staying in hotels along the way. Mary would point out the different waters and bridges where she would reminisce about where she and her husband would fish and boat.

I use the analogy of the game of life to be somewhat of a chessboard. You could either be the king on the board or the pawn. At about the age of 60, we start to look around at our chessboard of life. Where are we on the board? What does our financial health look like, our medical health, and what about our personal health? We look at our children, friends, retirement plans.

It is here that we value family even more; especially during a personal medical crisis. And we realize how important having a few good friends are. They can help us thwart loneliness and isolation especially when life throws us curve balls.

Change can always be good… if we keep a good outlook, remain connected, keep a sense of humor and remain flexible. I find that it is very important to pray every day, and be grateful for what I have.

So, Mom and I did arrive in CT, August 30 2020. As we drove up my driveway, she looked up at the "Tree of Heaven" in our yard where her husband had committed suicide and said "Nancy, did Dad die in October?" I said, "No, Mom, he died August 31, 2017, 3 years ago tomorrow."

Mom died October 12, 2020 of a ruptured brain aneurysm. This was not in our plans but we were so grateful she was with all of us during such a perilous time. Change is the only constant we have!

Durable Medical Equipment- What is it? (DME)

Any equipment such as a semi-electric bed with side rails or a wheelchair are called durable medical equipment (DME). Medicare Part B and Medicare Advantage Plans do cover this equipment if it is medically necessary and obtained from an approved supplier. Your HCP has to indicate in the medical record of the equipment's medical necessity and send an order to a medical supply company.

You can actually get many medical items from some websites, such as Facebook Marketplace: but remember, it has been used and will need careful inspection. A new company has emerged called "Wheel It Forward."

It is an on-line not-for-profit DME lending library in CT that is expanding into other states and is coming to a town near you. There is a National Directory called GotDME.org to find free places to borrow DME.

"It is a known fact that the average piece of DME has a lifespan of over five years but is used for only four months. The lightly used equipment ends up in garages, attics and basements. If you were to buy this equipment, it is 3 3 x higher than out-of-pocket costs for prescription drugs. Combine that with high deductible insurance plans and this equipment is unaffordable for many, even in the middle class. "Borrow rather than buy" says the website.

This directory supplies wheelchairs, knee scooters, hospital beds, rollators, shower safety equipment and more. Any lending closet can join this site so that people in your community can find you. It is in the early stages but please check it out. You can also join the email for updates.

I went to the library in Bridgeport, CT and was able to give a small donation to borrow a cleaned and inspected transfer tub chair, cane and knee scooter. I am to return them within 3 months once the equipment is no longer needed. This was a perfect situation for my family.

I had a patient who revised his home so that he no longer needed a stair lift. I had a patient miles away who needed it. I connected them both and a volunteer installed the system for the family. The daughters were able to take their mom to the beach by getting her down the stairs on the new stairlift, and into a wheelchair. They were most grateful since the stairlift used to be a purchase-only item costing people thousands of dollars. Now there are companies that rent the stairlift by the month.

One trick I have learned to cushion bed rails is to take two "noodles" that we use to float in water, and cut a slit down from one end to another. You can now just wrap the noodle around the railings. Use different colors to spice up the hospital bed!

There is more than one type of wheelchair if your mom is unable to support her head, or has difficulty sitting upright. This special wheelchair called a tilt-in-space wheelchair can be customized based on weight and body habitus. A rehabilitation center can fit the person for this special chair. It will take a few months to have the wheelchair made. Special devices can be customized such as arm rests for a paralyzed arm, and leg supports.

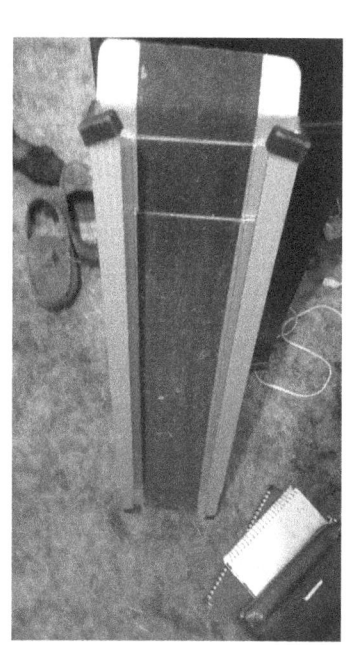

Foot drop is when the foot drops forward as a result of nerve injury or from muscle or nerve disorders causing difficulty walking. The muscles that support the top of the foot are weakened. One way to help support feet in a hospital bed is to apply a board to the end of the bed. The board flexes the feet, while the person lies in bed. Flop stop is an orthotic device that attaches to the shoe and behind the heel to support the foot from dropping when walking. Special shoes and braces can be fitted to the leg with the foot drop.

Ramps are now made to be portable and adjustable so you can change their length should you need to take a wheelchair-bound person down steps other than the home. The good part about this is you do not have to have a ramp built onto your house, which can get pricey depending on the length installed.

Elder and Caregiver Abuse

When we speak of abuse, it can take many forms. The first type of abuse is verbal abuse. It is evident by yelling, cursing or belittling someone. This could be done by the caregiver or by the patient. The evidence of anger can be a result of depression or dementia. For the patient, it has been found that if she was argumentative and difficult at a younger age, she will become more so as she ages with dementia.

Physical abuse is sometimes hard to determine since many of my patients have multiple bruises from fragile skin. I do watch the patient's reaction to the caregiver: does she look withdrawn or scared, not talking as if afraid. Episodes of falls, fractures and frequent hospital admissions may indicate some form of abuse. Families do install "nanny cams" to watch their parents at home while they are being cared for by an aide, just for peace of mind. They allow visibility of your mother's activities from another location. She is able to see how the aide and her mom spend their day together.

Neglect is another area of abuse. If I find the under garment soaked with urine, as if it has been on for many hours, I suspect neglect. Before making any assumptions, I ask how many times a day is the undergarment changed and is there any problems with changing it more often. Sometimes the reason it is not changed is that the caregiver needs someone to help her, or funds are limited to buy an adequate supply. Depending on the reason, I help solve the problem to avoid what may look like neglect.

If I feel there is concern about the patient's care such as non-compliance with medications for example, the patient is not taking insulin; or much discord in the home that appears harmful to the caregiver or the patient, I may refer to Adult Protective Services to make a home visit to determine how to help them.

Fall Prevention

Falling over the age of 60 has long-term negative implications on one's health. Broken bones can change your quality of life if there is poor healing or chronic pain. A more serious fall is when a head hits the floor, as it could lead to brain injuries. The chance of another fall is great after the first one. And usually, the person is afraid of falling again, so may reduce their activity. When this happens, the person becomes deconditioned and weak making falling even more predictable.

If the person is on a blood thinner and has a history of falling, it is important to discuss with your HCP the possibility of stopping this medication if the risk outweighs the benefit. The chance for serious bleeding increases when the person has a history of falling and is taking Coumadin or other blood thinners.

When I saw my patients at a regular visit, I always asked if she has had a recent fall. When one of my patients fall, I'd ask why or how? Does she remember what happened? Did she have a story about tripping on something, or was she dizzy? Did she forget to use her walker? Was she wearing poor-fitting shoes, or did she slip on a rug?

My father was having multiple falls but did not remember what happened. His wife was not home to witness them. First, he hit his head when falling in the kitchen while making a sandwich. He was taken to the hospital and found to have a small head bleed. He was sent home, then a week later, he fell in the driveway getting the mail. His blood work did not indicate he had anemia; his blood pressure was not dropping when he stood up (orthostatic hypotension), and he did not say he got dizzy and fell.

Then we had his 90th birthday party at a restaurant. While blowing out the candles, he fainted in his chair while his seven children and grandchildren were around him. I checked his pulse, and it was around 20 beats a minute. 911 was called, and he was transferred to the hospital and found to need a pacemaker. We picked up the birthday cake, brought it to the hospital and we all celebrated his birthday there. If there are no symptoms before the fall, or the is no recall of what happened, think low heart rate and the possible need for a pacemaker.

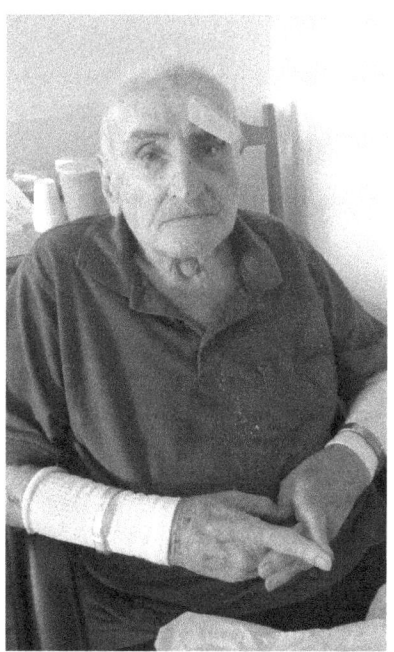

Fall prevention checklist for inside the home:

- Remove all loose wires, cords and throw rugs
- Keep floors free of clutter
- Remove raised doorway thresholds
- Be sure all carpets and area rugs have skid-proof backing or are tacked to the floor

- Do not use slippery wax on bare floors
- Install grab bars on the bathroom and hallway walls
- Keep stairwells well lit, with light switches at the top and the bottom
- Use night-lights in hallways and bathroom
- Consider installing clap on, clap off lights that are easy to turn on at night
- Move items that you use a lot to lower shelves but above waist level
- Keep a flashlight (with new batteries) and cell phone near your bed
- Wear low-heeled shoes that fit well and give your feet support. The soles should be non-skid.
- Check shoes regularly for wear, and replace as needed
- Do not wear socks without shoes on wood floors
- If you are using a cane, put a 4-way prong device that allows the cane to stand on its own for sturdiness

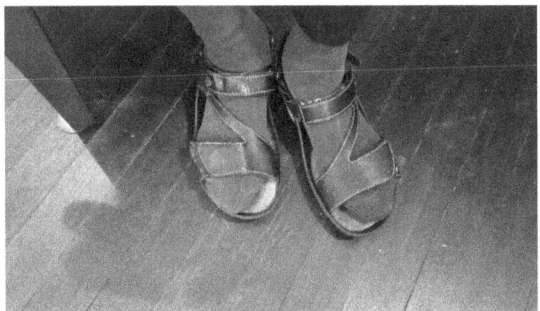

supportive sandals with backs- safe!

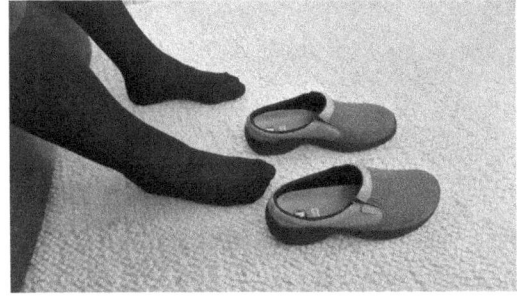

slippers with closed backs- safe!

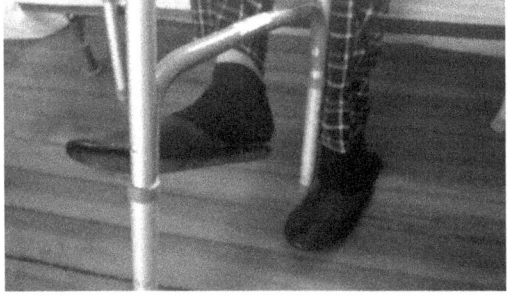

slippers with opened backs- not safe!

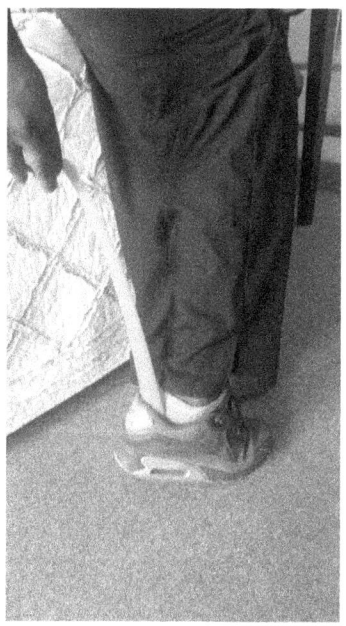

Long shoe horn helps with applying shoes independently

People wear shoes that have worn backs on them because they could not bend down to pull the back of the shoe over their foot. Essentially, these shoes become like slippers and can easily fall off. Get a long shoe horn, so the person does not have to reach down very far to put his shoes on correctly. Consider using the socks with the skids on the bottom if you cannot find safe slippers. (You know, the ones you get from the hospital when you are having a procedure.)

Fall prevention checklist for outside the home:

- Be careful on steps leading to front or rear doors
- Use a shoulder bag, fanny pack or backpack to leave hands free
- Wear warm boots with rubber soles for more solid footing
- Avoid wearing flip flops or open back shoes when the weather is bad
- Look carefully at floor surfaces in public buildings, which may be slippery
- Stop at curbs and check height before stepping up or down

FALL PREVENTION

- Wear glasses for better visual acuity
- Use a walker or cane as needed, especially in nasty weather
- Cover porch steps with gritty, weatherproof paint
- Install handrails on both sides of porch steps
- Walk on the grass when the sidewalks are slippery.

Preventing falls in the bathtub

- Install grab bars and non-skid mats inside and outside the shower or tub, and near the toilet and sinks
- Use shower chairs and bath benches
- Use a hand-held shower head that will allow you to sit while showering
- Get into the tub or shower by putting the weaker leg in first. Get out of a tub or shower with your strong side first
- Repair loose toilet seats and consider getting a raised toilet seat, so it is easier to get off the toilet
- Consider getting a 3-in-1 commode to have near your bed to use at night
- Keep your bathroom door unlocked while you are in the shower

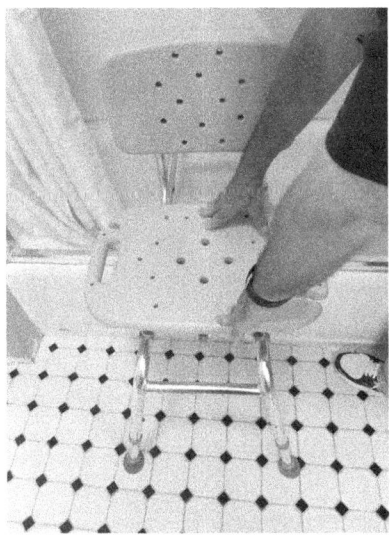 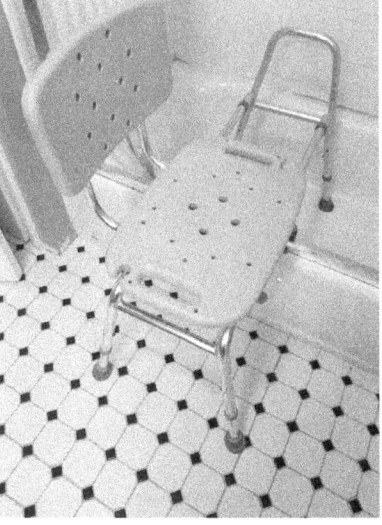 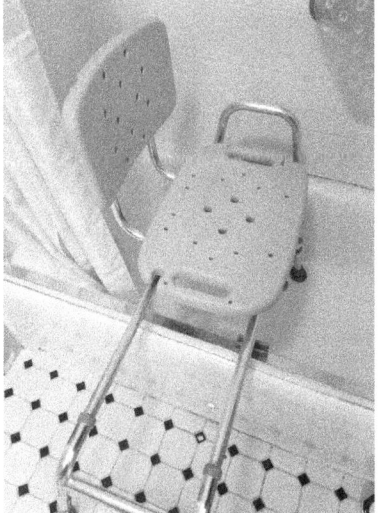

Versatility of a shower seat

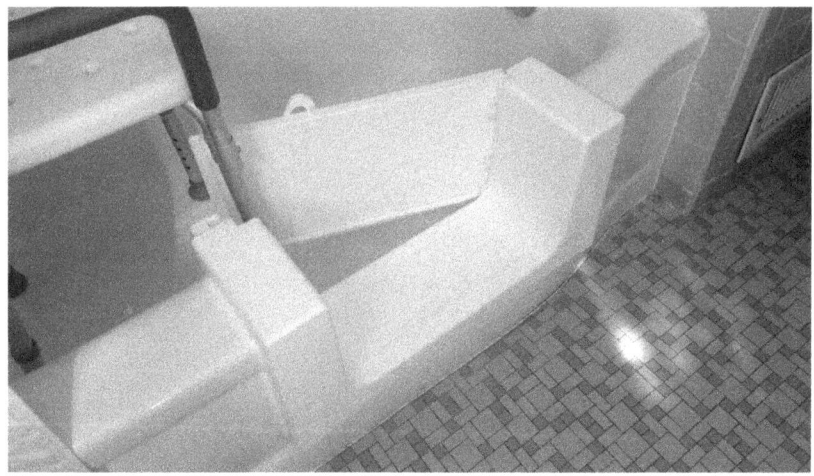

Easy alterations to an existing tub

Some good tips to reduce injury:

- Walking every day for 30 minutes can improve stamina and overall good muscle tone and conditioning.
- Take a Tai Chi class to learn better balance techniques (National Osteoporosis Foundation 6/2011)

There are home improvement contractors that are certified in home alterations for aging in place. They can widen doorways, put in ramps, railings, and alter showers to make them walk in with sit down benches, for example. Just google "Aging in Place Home Contractors." Look for a Certified Aging in Place Specialist (CAPS). The book "Moving in the Right Direction" by Bruce Nemovitz is an easy read for a better understanding about decluttering. You can also check out my video, "Do You Need to Declutter?" on my YouTube channel, Caregiver Success.

Lifeline, Life Alert, Medical Alert, etc. are all emergency devices worn on the wrist or around the neck. The person wearing the device pushes the button if there is an emergency, initiating a response from the local emergency room.

The ER calls the person to check what is wrong and activates the EMS system to send a police officer and a paramedic to the home, if necessary. These devices are different prices, so it is good to comparison shop. A cell phone is good to have on a person at all times with a speed dial for a family member and for 911.

Fire Prevention:
What to do in Case of a Fire

It is important to determine an escape plan should there be a fire. As your parent's condition changes, you need to change the plan for evacuation.

Absolutely no smoking in bed! One of my patients has small cigarette burns all over her bedspread since she spends most of her time in bed and is a chain smoker. I would tell her every time I visit her that she is in extreme danger of going up in flames.

- Do not smoke near an oxygen concentrator. If a spark is dropped near the machine, it can cause combustion and increase the power of a flame.
- Old homes have old electrical sockets, and overloading them with extension cords is dangerous.
- Remove clutter, so there is a clear path should you have to leave home immediately.
- Have a smoke and carbon dioxide detector on each floor of the home, and change the batteries every fall and spring.
- If you notice smoke from a room or a fire, get everyone out of the room and close the door. Place a wet towel at the base of the door and call 911.
- If the person is in a hospital bed, grab the bed sheet away from the bed, crank the bed to its lowest level. It is best if there are two people so each person can take a side of the sheet, gently lower the person to the floor, and pull him/her on the sheet down the hall and down the stairs.
- If the person can walk, remain calm and help her down the stairs, or out the back door.

- If an aide is there, she can call for help and assist you with the transport.
- It is also good to have an updated ABC fire extinguisher in the home. This extinguisher covers all types of fires.
- If you should actually catch on fire, remember the mnemonic: "Stop, Drop and Roll." Just drop to the floor and roll until the fire goes out. Do not go running out of the house as the fire will just get bigger.

Hand Washing/ Nail Care

It is important to keep fingernails short to reduce the spread of germs. Aides from agencies are not allowed to cut fingernails. The person who is bedridden, and cannot immerse her hands in water to wash them before eating, has an increased risk of getting sick from unclean hands and fingernails.

When their hands are under the covers, they sometimes scratch and can cause skin abrasions. If the person is confused, he may put hands down a soiled undergarment causing stool to adhere to the long nails. Using a baby wipe to clean the hands is not sufficient to assure cleanliness.

- As part of the daily cleaning, the patient can either be sat up in bed or wheeled to the bathroom sink.
- Provide a large bowl placed on a towel or use a basin that is flat on the bottom to prevent tipping.
- Fill it with warm, soapy water and place the hands in the water.
- Put on gloves, and wash the fingers, palms, and backs of hands. Wash the hands for at least one minute, using an orange stick to remove debris under the nails.
- Replace the water with clear warm water, and rinse the hands.
- Once the nails are soft and clean, they can be cut.

Hand Washing- How to Prevent the Spread of Germs

Don't you hate it when you are in a public bathroom and the person who comes out of the stall, walks right out of the bathroom after touching the bathroom doorknob? Germs are spread so easily this way.

HAND WASHING/ NAIL CARE

When you take care of someone, wearing gloves is NOT a replacement for washing hands. **Always** wash hands before and after glove use. Always wear gloves when touching any bodily secretions- mouth care, wound care, and changing undergarments. It will also good to wear gloves when bathing someone. Always wash the person's hands before meals.

Here are the simple steps for washing your hands:

You will need a soap dispenser or a bar of soap (as long as it is in a container that drains).

1. Wet your hands with warm water leaving the faucet running
2. Squirt a dispenser full of liquid soap in the palm of your hand
3. Wash between the fingers, palms, backs of the hands for a total of 20 seconds
4. While the water is running, rinse hands well to remove all soap
5. Dry with paper towels or a designated clean towel
6. Turn off the faucet with the paper towel
7. Use the paper towel on the doorknob to open the door
8. Toss the paper towel into the garbage while holding the door open with your elbow

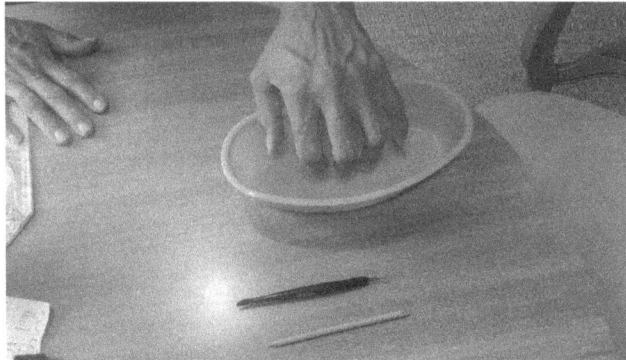
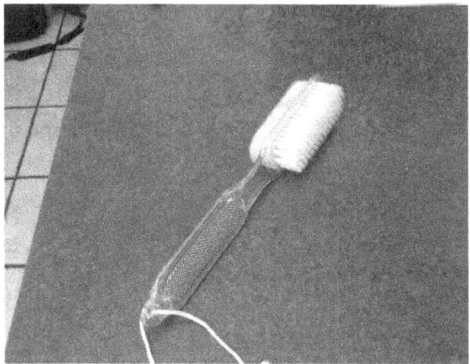

Emesis basin and orange stick for nail cleaning, nailbrush

Heat Safety Tips

Dehydration can be very dangerous for the elderly or frail person. It is important to have an air conditioner in at least one room where the person can stay, especially when it is 90 degrees or higher for 48 hours or more.

Offer less protein and more fruits and vegetables. Protein produces and increases metabolic heat, which causes water loss. Eat small meals, but eat often. Do not eat salty foods. Drink at least 2-4 ounces of water /hour during extreme heat, even if you do not feel thirsty. Avoid beverages containing alcohol or caffeine. If you do not live near your parent, have a neighbor periodically check in on him or her.

How to Take Vital Signs

It is a necessary proponent of care for the caregiver to be able to take vital signs on the patient. Vital signs include pain evaluation, oxygen saturation, temperature, pulse, respiration and blood pressure. By obtaining this basic information, the status of the patient can be objectively determined. Vital signs should be taken when the person is at rest and has not had anything to eat, drink or smoke for 30 minutes. Always remember to wash your hands before touching your patient and tell him what you are going to do.

Let's take this evaluation one by one. First how do you evaluate someone's pain?

If the person is alert and is a good historian then it can be somewhat easy. Otherwise, you would have to be very observant. If the person is not a good historian, look at the person's face as you touch various parts of the body to watch for grimacing or sounds of groaning. You would have to put together a story, such as any incidents that happened, when they happened, was there any bruising, or change in the person's ability to move an extremity.

If the person is alert and can tell you, ask:

Where is your pain?
What is the intensity of your pain?
What relieves your pain: position? Medications?
When did your pain start?
Does your pain come and go or is it all the time?
What aggravates your pain?
Does the pain radiate to another part of your body?

Be sure to record these findings in your daily logbook so you can keep track of the sequence of events, hence, the patient's medical story.

Oxygen Saturation is the "fraction of oxygen-saturated hemoglobin relative to total hemoglobin in the blood. If the saturation is below 80%, it can cause impaired mental function. The normal range is between 95-100%. If a person continues to have an oxygen level less than 88%, he may need to be on portable oxygen. You will need to buy an oximeter which can be purchased in any pharmacy.

How to obtain an oxygen saturation reading:

- Clean the tip of the index finger with an alcohol wipe
- Apply an oximeter (a meter that fits on the finger) to the tip of the index finger
- You will see a number appear on the screen
- Record the reading in your logbook
- Clean the device with an alcohol wipe after use

How to take a temperature:

Temperature can be taken orally, axillary (armpit) temporal (forehead), tympanic (ear) or rectally. Glass thermometers are no longer considered useful or safe. Because of the glass and the environmental exposure to mercury, the glass thermometer should be disposed of by putting it inside a disposable plastic container, pour kitty litter, dirt or sand around it filling the entire container and apply a tight lid. Dispose of it in the trash.

If the person is alert, use an oral digital thermometer. She would be able to follow directions. An oral temperature ranges from 97 to 99 degrees Fahrenheit. A fever is an oral temperature over 100 degrees Fahrenheit. (F).

How to take an oral temperature:

- Before use, wipe the thermometer tip that goes into the mouth with an alcohol wipe
- Use a disposable sheathe cover on the thermometer
- Tell the person to open his mouth
- Place the thermometer under the tongue
- Tell the person to close his mouth as you hold the thermometer in his mouth
- Wait for the beep sound
- Record the temperature reading in your logbook and write "oral" next to the reading
- Use an alcohol wipe to clean the tip of the thermometer

A normal axillary temperature is usually a degree **lower** than an oral temperature. It ranges from 96.6 F to 98 degrees F. You can use an oral thermometer to take an axillary temperature.

How to take an axillary temperature:

- Wipe the tip of the thermometer with an alcohol wipe
- Use a disposable sheathe cover on the thermometer
- Place the thermometer under the arm in the armpit area
- Have the person keep her arm close to her body until you hear a beep sound
- Record the reading in your logbook and write "axillary" next to the reading
- Use an alcohol wipe and clean the sensor of the thermometer

How to take a temporal temperature:

A temporal thermometer is a special thermometer that reads heat waves from the temporal artery

- Place the sensor head at the center of the forehead
- Slowly slide the thermometer across the forehead toward the top of the ear
- Stop when you reach the hairline
- Read the monitor and record in your logbook with "temporal" next to it
- When done, wipe the sensor with an alcohol wipe to clean it

A rectal temperature is taken when it is difficult to take a temperature any of the other ways. A rectal temperature is 0.5 to 1 degree **higher** than an oral temperature. Fever is defined as a rectal temperature over 100 degrees F. Once the thermometer is used rectally, it should not be used in the mouth or anywhere else.

How to take a rectal temperature:

- Place the person on his side
- Put a small amount of petroleum jelly on the tip of the thermometer probe
- Gently spread the buttock cheeks apart to visualize the rectum
- Gently place the thermometer probe in the rectum approximately 1 inch and hold it in place
- Wait for the beep and record the reading in your logbook writing "rectal" after it
- Clean the tip of the thermometer with an alcohol wipe

A tympanic thermometer measures using an infrared sensor to measure the temperature of energy radiating from the eardrum. The normal ear temperature for adults is 99.5 degrees F.

How to use a tympanic thermometer:

- Use a clean probe tip each time, and follow the manufacturer's instructions
- Tug gently on the top of the ear and pull it back
- Gently insert the thermometer to seal the ear canal
- Squeeze down the button on the device for one second
- Remove the thermometer and read the temperature
- Record the temperature in your logbook and write "ear" next to the reading
- Use warm water and mild detergent to clean the handset and base, dry and return to its case

Next, let's learn how to obtain a heart rate. Heart rate is the rate the heart is beating in 60 seconds. If the person seems to have an irregular heart rate, where you notice it is not a consistent beat, it is important to evaluate the heartbeat for one full minute; and if the heartbeat seems regular without beats skipping, you can measure it for just 15 seconds then multiply x 4 to get a heartbeat in 60 seconds.

A heart rate over 100 beats/ minute is called "tachycardia" and below 60, is called "bradycardia." Different heart rates can be caused by emotions, being a smoker, having pain, medications side effect, age and body position (standing up or lying down).

How to check a heart rate:

You do not need to have a stethoscope to check a heart rate. You will need a wristwatch to watch the seconds.

- Place your index and middle finger gently on the patient's wrist on the side of his thumb (do not use your thumb because it has a pulse of its own)

- When you feel the pulse, look at your watch second hand and begin counting the pulse for 15 seconds
- Multiply that number by 4 (for example, if you count 15 beats in 15 seconds x 4= 60 beats/minute.
- Record this reading in your logbook
- If the pulse feels irregular, count the beats for a full one minute to get an accurate reading, and record "irregular" next to the rate

Now we will learn how to obtain a respiratory rate. It is the number of breaths a person takes in one minute. The rate is measured when the person is at rest and involves counting the person's chest movement as it rises and falls, which indicates one breath. A normal respiratory rate for an adult at rest is 12-20 breaths/minute. A person will change their breathing pattern if you tell them what you are going to do.

How to check respiratory rate:

- Pretend that you are taking the person's pulse while looking at his chest for movement
- Watch the chest rise and fall
- Take note on your watch to count for 15 seconds
- One breath equals one rise and fall of the chest
- Count the breaths for 15 seconds, then multiply by 4
- You now have a respiratory rate for one minute
- Record it in your logbook

(Look under Section 2: Hypertension- Common in the Older Adult to learn how to take a proper blood pressure reading)

(Check out YouTube on Caregiver Success- "How to take Vital Signs")

Humor and Introspection- Time to laugh

It is healthy to embrace who you are, what you now look like as you age, and what makes you laugh. Humor is a tremendous stress reliever, and with laughing you release endorphins. Endorphins are hormones that help with immunity and reduces disease. The more you take things lighter and laugh, the better your outlook will be as well as your health.

As I wandered through literature, looking for information for this book, I found books about all sorts of views on aging. I must say, I have a good sense of humor. The important thing is knowing when it an appropriate time to laugh and get silly, and when not to. I am very in-tune with my patients. We know that getting old is not for sissies. One book given to me was "I'm New at Being Old" with art and narrative by Lucy Rose Fischer. It is very introspective with pictures of how the person felt about getting old and how she perceived how others treat the elderly.

Another book is: "In Dog Years I'm Dead" *Growing Old (Dis) Gracefully*, written by Carol Lynn Pearson. I dug it out and was laughing hysterically by page 10. Watching a funny movie, telling jokes, seeing friends who make you laugh and smile, are actually a way to get you to feel good.

One day I went to visit Mildred F. She was one of my favorite patients. At 98, she was sharp and witty, but Parkinson's disease limited her mobility. I told her I was having a birthday, so she wanted to give me something to wear there. Her husband found a yellow feathered boa with a crown that was given to her for one of her parties. I could not consider taking it, but she was happy to wear it for me during our visit. She always made me laugh.

Hurricane Safety Tips

How to be prepared for your older parent:

- If your parent lives in a hurricane zone and you are not nearby, have them prepare for a hurricane
- Make arrangements for life support equipment, such as oxygen. Get portable tanks that do not require electricity
- Identify a friend or family member from a non-threatened area who will be kept informed about your family's plans
- Plan what to do with the pets
- Inventory personal property; safely secure all records and valuable documents in a watertight place
- Have emergency cash or traveler's checks saved
- Have materials to protect doors and windows

Prepare a Hurricane Evacuation Kit:

- First Aid Kit
- A two-week supply of medicine
- Blankets or sleeping bags
- Extra clothing
- Personal items, including books
- Valid ID
- Checkbook, cash, credit cards, ATM cards

Long-Term Care Insurance- Have you considered it?

Long-term care insurance is having coverage that will pay for assisted living, nursing home care or home health care if you should be unable to care for yourself because of a chronic condition or disability. For those who cannot afford long-term care, Medicaid and reverse mortgage is an option.

Policies purchased in the 1990s may have premiums that you can no longer afford, making the risk for losing the policy greater when you need the policy the most.

Now that insurers have had data collected from decades of claims, premiums should be less volatile in the future. At this time, when buying a policy, the risk is included in the premium. The carriers thought that people would drop the policies as they got older, but instead, people are living longer. They are not necessarily living healthier. There were higher claims made and many of the insurance companies opted out of the market.

Short-term care insurance is similar to the long-term care insurance policies, but there is usually a cap of one year to use the benefits. They may be a better option for seniors that are not eligible for long-term coverage.

Health savings accounts (HSA)

Many places of employment have wellness programs, because if the employee is well, he shows up to work, is productive and saves them money on medical claims. When my husband was employed, there was a wellness website, and every time I would listen to different subjects, like how to eat better, or ways to exercise in front of the TV, I would accrue money that is put into my HSA. This money is tax-deferred and is banked for medical costs. We have a very high deductible health insurance plan, so this helps out. Long-term insurance premiums can be paid from an HSA.

Discuss your options with a certified financial planner to help you with long term goals. The younger age you decide on a policy, the less the premium will be to carry over the years.

Money Matters- What is a Personal Money Manager?

As our parent's age, it becomes more difficult for some to manage their daily financial transactions. There have been instances where the children are at odds with each other over their parents' finances; and unfortunately, can cause a division in the family.

If you are looking for someone to help your parents with their finances, help pay bills, manage their mail, help budget, keep track of medical and other insurance claims, consider getting a personal money manager. They can double-check their accounts to make sure there is no suspicious activity.

This field is fairly new, and financial caregivers come from a variety of backgrounds and expertise. It is important to start by asking people you trust, such as an accountant or an attorney you know. You can also check out the American Association of Daily Money Managers, which is a national organization with over 800 members. They subscribe to a code of ethics and standard of practice, requiring disclosure of any conflict of interest.

My colleague, Karen Rosenberg Caccavo is a personal money manager, also called "financial caregiver." Do not get this title mixed up with Power of Attorney, which is a legal designation. She has blogs you can watch on her website: https://personalmoneymanager.net

It is great to think ahead when it comes to working with an aging parent. If you see that your mother is getting more forgetful with taking care of financial matters, it helps to step in early on, perhaps get your name on her checkbook and ask her if you can see a lawyer making you the financial POA. She may also ask you to be her health care proxy. It is less threatening and scary for Mom if you do both medical and financial at the same time.

The home deed can be turned over from the bank to a child, taking it out of the parent's name. If there is more than one child in the family, your mother may pick the one that she feels is the most responsible and understands her wishes the best. This decision can be difficult because feelings could be hurt. I have been involved in court cases to advocate for the elderly person as the children fought over their parent's assets.

I talk with my families to think ahead, as their parents get older, because once the person needs help with their finances, the banks are legally bound to the customer, and will not work with the child, even if your mother has become unable to do her finances. As a nurse practitioner, I am unable to deem someone incompetent or incapacitated even if it is evident the person has some form of dementia. A psychiatrist and an internist have to make this diagnosis.

If your mother needs to get Medicaid, it could take up to 5 years to get her cleared from owning property. This action of changing home ownership can assure aging in place since aides could be hired using Medicaid. In other states, if your mother has Medicaid, she is evaluated by a nurse who determines how much aide services she needs. Sometimes she has a 12-hour aide during the day and another aide at night; or a live-in aide.

In New York State, there is a Medicaid program called CDPAP, which stands for "Consumer Directed Personal Assistance Program." It is a great idea because many caregivers have to quit their jobs or pay for private care while they are working, and this can be difficult financially.

Depending on what state you live in, you should explore what is available. Call Medicaid, Office of the Aging, speak with a social worker; and consider seeing an elder lawyer to sort through the legalities. Ask what your friends are doing to get care; this is the time to network and "get your ducks in a row."

Mouth Care

Can you imagine what it would be like if you never brushed your teeth again? Food left in the mouth leads to bad breath, bad taste, gingivitis (infected gums), black or breaking teeth, jaw bone weakness, etc. The plaque would build up around the teeth, and gums would start to bleed. Some of what I have seen is just from neglect. The person could be clean, dressed and hair washed, but when I examine their mouths, I see food particles and swollen gums. Just because we are getting older, does not mean we have to lose our teeth!

Even if the person has no teeth, it is important to perform some kind of mouth care twice a day. Dentures should be soaked at least 4 hours every 24 hours in a denture cleaner that you can get over-the-counter. By doing this, it helps to keep the lining of your mouth healthy.

A toothette is a sponge on a stick that can be dipped in a mouth wash such as Biotene. I like this product because patients like the taste and it can improve moisture in the mouth. It especially works well on a bedbound patient who cannot get to the sink.

More than one toothette can be used to remove any food trapped in the lower gum areas. In addition, using a toothbrush with toothpaste for brushing the roof of the mouth, any remaining teeth, and the tongue! This is the time to look around the mouth for any problems, such as candidiasis or leukoplakia (oral cancer).

Another good device is a tongue scraper. It actually scrapes debris off of the tongue. It may help you determine if the person has candidiasis. Candidiasis (also known as thrush) is a coating of creamy white material (looks like milk) on the tongue or patches inside the mouth. The tongue can be red, painful and smooth. There could be cracking at the corners of the mouth. If you notice that the patient is not eating and losing weight, make sure to look at their tongue for candidiasis. This condition can be easily treated with an anti-fungal agent.

A scraping using a culturette (a specimen-collecting device) from the lab can find out for sure what it is. People with diabetes, taking certain antibiotics, a weakened immune system, and those with cancer tend to develop this condition. The treatment is Mycelex troches that can be sucked on up to 5 a day for 2 weeks. This may be hard for some people to do so a pill called Diflucan (fluconazole) can be given instead.

Leukoplakia is another condition that can be found in the mouth. It appears as a gray or white patch on the person's tongue, the floor of the mouth or on the inside of the cheek. It is not usually painful, but sometimes sensitive to spicy foods, heat or touch. The dentist is usually the person to find this condition. A biopsy is needed to rule out oral cancer. This involves taking a small sample of the tissue to examine in the lab.

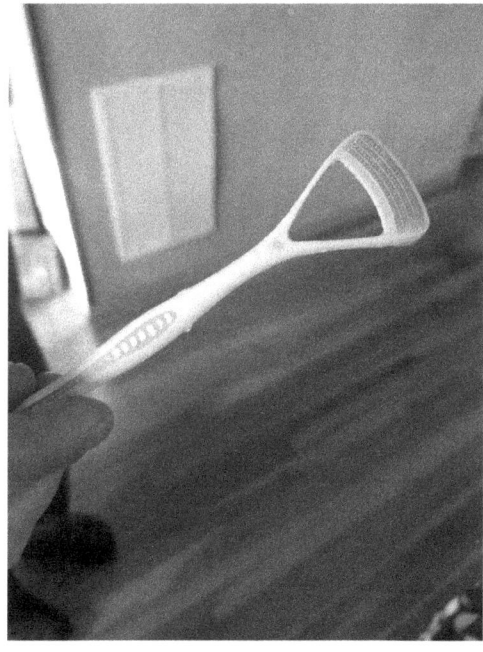

Tongue scraper

MOUTH CARE

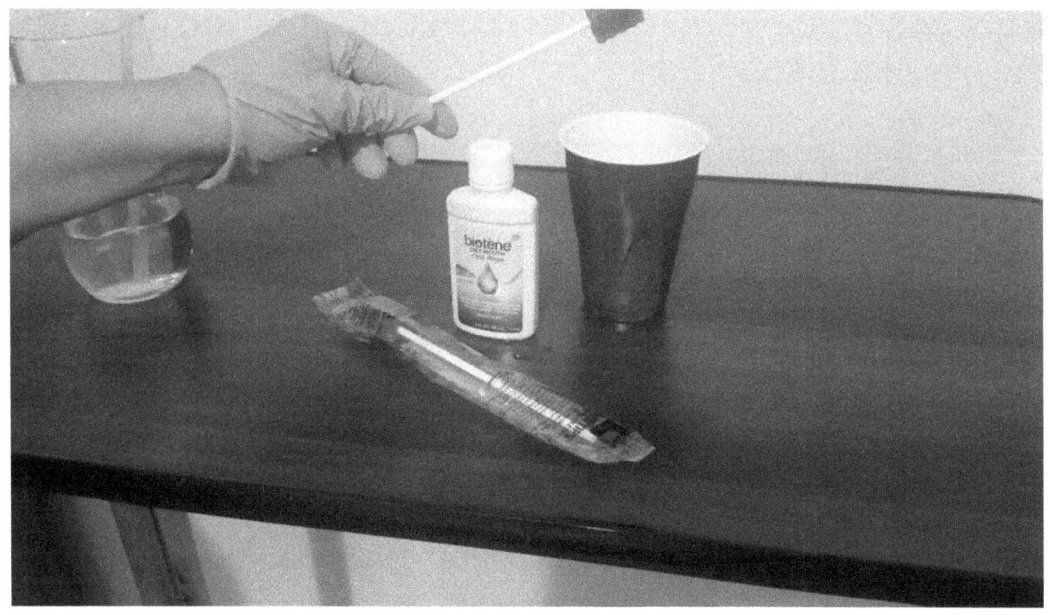

Mouth care items

There are many portable medical services for the home of which you can find online. For one is a dentist. He/she cannot perform everything he does in the office, but the care can be adequate in the home. Patients can lie in a chair recliner with a floor lamp nearby for good lighting, and have a good exam with a dental cleaning from a dentist. Dentures and partial plates can be repaired or sized, and brought back from his office for a fitting.

Some dentists do not take Medicare, however. You may want to consider getting some type of dental insurance so you can have regular care that is not that costly. Medicaid does cover most dental care. If dental care is extensive, such as a tooth extraction, an ambulette can transport the person to the office, with work done while in the wheelchair. A medical clearance would need to be done by your HCP.

The risk for cavities happens at all ages. It is recommended to have a dental exam at least once a year. And do not wait until you have pain! As we age, the nerves inside the teeth become smaller and less sensitive. By the time you feel pain from a cavity, it may be too late, and you may lose your tooth.

Here are some tips from the American Dental Association (ADA) for the over 60 folks:

- Brush teeth in the morning and in the evening. If you have to brush someone else's mouth, consider getting an electric toothbrush to make it easier, and use fluoride toothpaste. This device makes a noise if you are pressing too hard on the teeth, which tells you to lighten the pressure
- Replace your toothbrush, or toothbrush head, every 3-4 months
- Buy products that have the ADA seal of approval, which has been around since 1931
- Use individual flossers to make it easier to get between someone else's teeth. Floss twice a day, if possible
- Drink water with fluoride at any age to prevent tooth decay.
- It is never too late to quit smoking. Check out smokefree.gov about ways to help you quit

When you see the dentist bring:

- A list of your medications, including vitamins, over-the-counter, and herbal remedies.
- A list of medical conditions and allergies
- Important phone numbers and names of HCPs
- Information about medical contacts
- Your dentures, even if you don't wear them

The Healing Power Music has on Seniors

Music has been known to be a powerful way to connect with an aging adult. An otolaryngologist from Johns Hopkins explains "There are few things that stimulate the brain the way music does....If you wan to keep your brain engaged through the aging process, listening to or playing music is a great tool. It provides a total brain workout."

Research has found that music therapy can provide incredible benefits:

- Improving language and speech skills
- Lowering stress and anxiety levels
- Improving sleep quality
- Helping with memory
- Boosting creativity
- Reducing cognitive decline
- Improving sleep quality

So, turn on your favorite music to lift your spirits and begin dancing, even from a chair. Long-term dancing can improve coordination, flexibility and endurance. If you or your loved one plays an instrument, encourage him to pick it up and play a tune!

Since the internet, there are apps on your phone and YouTube where you can find everything from Disco to Wall Pilates, to chair exercises to Yoga. Whatever your favorite music is: Rock n' Roll, Classical, Country, etc. put on the music and begin to move. You can dance from your bed, your wheelchair or standing.

Begin with moving your neck, arms and move down to your feet. It starts the day with a smile and helps with joint mobility. The more you move, the better you will be health-wise!

Pets- what they mean to us

Having a pet, be it a cat, dog or even a pig, helps a person who may live alone to have companionship. A pet gives a person a sense of purpose, someone to love and care for. The pet becomes a person. It is a fact that a pet is kissed more than a significant other! It is also a fact that depression can be reduced and people live longer if he has a pet.

I had a funny experience at one of my patient's homes. One day, when visiting a patient, I heard a snorting. Jessica proceeded to bring "Oscar Chubbs" the pet pig, up the stairs to meet me. She says the pig, and his brother, sleep with her children at night. They are very affectionate and clean.

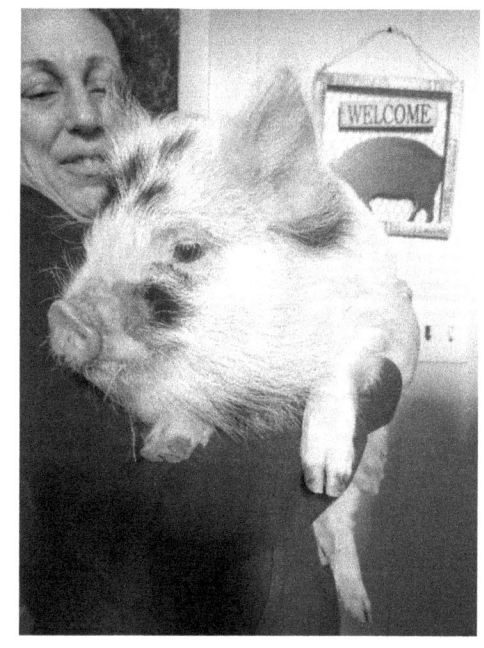

The pet industry has exploded. You can buy almost anything on line for your pet: clothes, treats, toys, gadgets, travel items, etc. They even have fitted life vests for boating. It seems our children in their 20s and 30s are deciding to wait on having children and are replacing them lovingly with dogs and cats. The money spent on Vet appointments can be astronomical. Sometimes the person forgoes his own medical needs in order to pay pet bills.

The loss of a pet that someone has had for years can be devastating. People grieve a pet like the loss of a long-time friend. My children had a dog named Kodiak who was 2 years old when we got him. My daughter, Chelsea was 9 at the time. Kodiak lived for 17 more years.

Chelsea was now 26. The dog was a big part of her life. She now has a teacup Pomeranian named Bella and recently added a husky named Bucky.

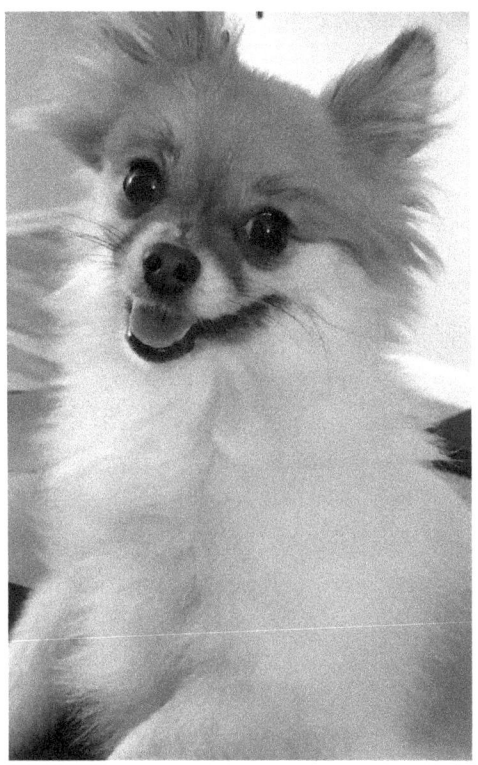

Small pets can be can be the reason for a tragic fall or injury. If your dog gets underfoot while you are walking with a rolling walker, you can get entangled and have a dangerous fall. So, be careful and always look where you are walking! They sure are cute though.

There are actually mechanical pets, such as cats that purr or move their heads or tails when they are patted. This type of pet is lifelike and is easy for a caregiver to have because there is no maintenance. My patient had dementia and loved his mechanical cat.

Podiatry-Having a Professional Take Care of your Feet

One of the people I networked into my home care practice was a traveling podiatrist. He was important to my patients because many of them needed foot care. I would call him when patients had problems like bunions, corns and infections. He visited the patients every 9 weeks (as per Medicare) for nail clipping and sooner if we called him with a problem.

Nails are to be cut straight across unless the nail is too thick. The corners, then, may need to be cut. A podiatrist will check feet for circulation, rashes, arthritis, injury, swelling and pressure areas. Part of the visit, especially for a diabetic, is to check for neuropathy and any wear from the person's shoes.

A microfilament is a small flexible stick-like structure used to test a single point of pressure. It can help determine if there is a lack of sensation when touching different parts of the toes and feet.

Fungal toenails (onychomycosis) are not treated with Lamisil on the older adult due to possible effects on the liver. Terbinafine is the drug of choice. A podiatrist would grind down the nail and treat it with additional products called Penlac nail polish, or Vick's VapoRub.

If there is a suspicion of a fractured toe, we would order a home x-ray for an accurate diagnosis. If one of the middle toes are found to be fractured, the treatment of choice is to "buddy tape" it. Taking surgical tape, you wrap the middle toe to the adjacent toe, giving the fractured toe stability to heal. It will take about 6 weeks for a fracture to heal. If the first or 5th toe is fractured, just wrap that individual toe with Coban.

What is a Prosthetist/ Orthotist?

A prosthetist is a specialist who customizes limbs, braces and shoes. If a person has hammertoes, or deformed feet, regular shoes may not fit. Ill-fitting shoes lead to foot sores and more deformities. Medicare, unfortunately, does not pay for these shoes unless a prescription is obtained from an endocrinologist or podiatrist. Even so, the shoes may not be totally covered. A pair of shoes can cost up to $500, and with custom inlays, another $400.

You can google where to get customized foot wear. Foot Lab, for example will cast, measure, scan and photograph your feet to create a 3D computer model before sending it to a manufacturing facility. Shoes are built to exact measurements so the fit is very accurate.

Power Outage- Be Prepared!

If your mom has any device that requires electricity for her care, such as an oxygen concentrator, tube feeding machine, or nebulizer, they should be registered with your local electric company. Usually, a form is completed by your HCP indicating that your mom is truly on a device that is life-sustaining or she would need to use it 12 hours a day.

If your mom is on oxygen, ask for your provider to order back-up portable tanks. Also, watch that the tanks are always half-full especially when there are warnings of a power outage. If it looks as if the outage is going to last more than a few days, consider moving your loved one out of her home with the oxygen tanks.

Have a list of emergency numbers readily available. It is also good to have a battery-operated radio, flashlight, and a supply of batteries on hand.

Keep an emergency supply of water, medications and non- perishable foods handy. If you have refrigerated items, keep the refrigerator closed for several hours to assure your foods remain cold. Consider filling plastic containers with water, leaving an inch of space inside each one- this will help keep food cold longer if the power goes out.

Consider buying a generator and follow the rules for using it outside your residence. It is best to have it installed by a qualified electrician.

If you have other questions, you can call your local Fire and Emergency Services in your county.

Rehabilitation

Many of us are quite familiar with therapy such as physical therapy, occupational and speech therapy. Either we have experienced this care, or one of our family members or friends have. My husband loved to play basketball. When he was 42 years old, he was running after a loose ball and pivoted sliding on a sandy surface causing him to fall to the ground with excruciating pain of his right knee. He got up with the help of friends, returned to work thinking he had a sprain, but the pain was getting worse. Steve is not a good patient- he didn't try Aleve or icing the knee.

The knee was feeling better after 3 days but was not feeling the same, and felt unstable to stand on. Then he saw his PCP who thought it was a sprain, so no x-rays were ordered. He continued to go on with work and home life and actually went back to playing basketball with the return of excruciating pain in the right knee. He went back to his PCP who then recommended Steve see an orthopedic surgeon where he had an x-ray and MRI of the right knee, with a diagnosis of a torn medial meniscus and severed ACL. He had a reconstruction of the ACL and repair of the meniscus.

For the next 6 months, Steve was in intensive therapy first in a rehabilitation center, and then at a gym for another 3 months. For the first two weeks, he was on a machine for 18 hours at night for range of motion. He had to wear a leg brace for 3 months to prevent injury. He was able to return to basketball 7 months after the surgery. He says playing basketball again "it was a mental thing" where he was afraid of getting re-injured. He had to commit time and effort in order to get back to a normal state. He was a young man going through this so you can imagine how an elderly person feels when they have to have surgery such as a hip replacement.

Steve, my husband, had his left hip replaced by Mako Robotics surgery last month. He did not want a walker and would not rent the ice machine for the leg. His orthopedist told me he was a "one look." This means that one look at his x-ray showed the erosion and deterioration of the left hip, warranting a total hip replacement. The surgery involved an anterior incision only a 4-inch long. Above this area was a staple line where the robotic probes were inserted. Steve was told he has no limitations. The hip replacement will take two years for total healing.

Some people are better patients than others. On day 4, I found Steve out mowing the lawn on the tractor! He suffered the consequences of taking "no limitations" too far. His upper thigh became very painful and swollen. He had to rest for 2 days to recover. It was not easy being his caregiver.

(See my YouTube videos at Caregiver Success on the days after Mako Total Hip Surgery)

One of my patients was having balance issues and was unsteady with the walker around her home. I ordered physical therapy, and when I went back two months later, she was walking safely and without any signs of imbalance. She had a smile on her face and looked proud that she was able to improve her abilities at home and prevent falls.

What is Rehabilitation?

Rehabilitation is a treatment or treatments designed to help the process of recovery from injury, illness, or disease to as normal a condition as possible. Rehabilitation can be ongoing for maintenance reasons and to prevent reversal of movement of joints.

Purpose

The main purpose of rehabilitation is to help bring back or restore function, be it physical, sensory, and /or mental, that was lost due to injury, illness or disease. Rehabilitation assists to compensate for a function that has been lost, such as due to amputation, arthritis, cancer, heart disease, neurological changes from Parkinson's or stroke, and brain injuries.

Any one person may need rehabilitation more than once in their lifetime, based on changes in health or body status. Maintaining function is the key, so following a daily program could be very beneficial to continue with a better quality of life and to prevent deterioration or de-conditioning of muscles. When you lose function, you lose the ability to take care of yourself.

Part of the rehabilitation may be a change in the physical environment, such as making a walk- in bathroom shower or adding rails in the hallways. It may be the use of a walker or a leg brace. Each program is tailored to an individual's needs. The Rehabilitation team consists of PT, OT, ST (if applicable), nurses, physiatrists (physical medicine) psychologists, prosthetists and social workers.

In order to get therapy, a licensed health provider such as a physician, physician's assistant or nurse practitioner would need to order it. Services are provided through either a certified home health agency (CHHA) or rehab program. I worked with a few different facilities that do house calls. Once the therapy starts, we keep in touch to discuss the person's progress. It is truly a team approach that helps the person get well.

What are the differences between the types of rehabilitation therapies? Let's review them.

Physical therapy (PT)

The educational requirement to become a physical therapist is a Master's degree from an accredited program. Physical therapists now are required to go on to get a doctoral degree, which takes about three years to complete.

The goal behind physical therapy is to restore the use of muscles, bones, and the nervous system by using cold, heat, massage, ultrasound, exercise, and other techniques, rather than by drugs and surgery. The physical therapist assesses and addresses various components of mobility and seeks to improve the quality of life.

These components may include general fatigue, weakness, tight muscles, dizziness, and poor balance, falls and fear of falling. They also work with edema management, pain and decreased endurance.

In the home, the treatments are more limited. If the person would benefit from more extensive treatment, he may need to go to a rehabilitation center, where he can receive other therapies as well. They start their assessment by taking a comprehensive patient history (past injuries, surgeries, medications, prognosis, psychosocial and home situation). The physical therapist is like a coach, who sets up a customized goal-patient-focused program.

The program can change depending on the illness or injuries as well as the person's response to therapy. Medications can affect balance and other physiological responses to exercise, so it is important that the physical therapist reviews them.

Occupational therapy (OT)

Occupational therapy helps the person to regain the ability to do normal tasks that they were used to doing every day (activities of daily living); such as dressing, bathing, grooming, meal preparation, medication management, and home maintenance. These therapists work mostly with the upper extremities and help with adaptive equipment, such as reachers, special utensils/ plates for eating, among many other things.

They can go to the patient's home and analyze what the person's abilities are in their environment. It may mean moving furniture, putting in ramps, etc. They help with transfer methods for getting out of the home and car. Online you can check out Aging in Place contractors who can adapt counters in the kitchen, shower stalls, outdoor stairs with ramps, stair lifts, etc.

Speech Therapy (ST)

They assess, diagnose, and treat various components of one's speech, language, social communication, cognition, and swallowing. They work with patients to improve the volume of speech and quality; work with reading and writing, and ability to safely tolerate food, liquids, and medications. They work with cognitive deficits such as memory, attention, executive function and orientation.

If the person is coughing when swallowing, a speech therapist should be asked to evaluate their swallowing technique to assure they are not going to aspirate when drinking fluids.

How to Care for your Respiratory Equipment

A Respiratory Therapist (RT) is a specialized professional who has graduated from a respiratory therapy program accredited by the Commission on Accreditation for Respiratory Care. They are trained in the assessment and treatment of patients with both acute and chronic dysfunction of the cardiopulmonary system.

When a person is ordered to start oxygen and other respiratory equipment, the vendor will send the respiratory therapist to the home to instruct the patient and the family how to use and care for the equipment. If you have any questions about this, you can call your vendor who delivered your equipment so that the respiratory therapist can come out or troubleshoot on the phone.

How to Use and Take Care of Your Nebulizer

Read over the care instructions that comes with your nebulizer, and do not discard them.

After each treatment, do the following:

- Wash your hands
- Take the cup apart that you put the medicine in (see instructions below)
- Rinse the mask or mouthpiece with warm water for at least 30 seconds
- Do not wash the nebulizer tubing or the compressor
- Shake off excess water and place parts on a clean towel for air-drying
- Re-assemble the system and turn on the compressor for a few seconds for drying

Once a week:

- Consult your owner's manual for instructions for care of the equipment
- You can soak the disassembled cup, in one part distilled white vinegar/three parts hot water for one hour (not the mask, tubing or compressor)
- Rinse the parts with warm water, shake off excess water, and allow to air-dry on a clean towel
- Reassemble the pieces and tubing and turn on the compressor briefly for drying
- The nebulizer mask should NEVER go through the dishwasher
- Keep the nebulizer covered and in a clean place until next use
- Nebulizer tubing should be changed every 6 months

Changing Nebulizer Filters

It is strongly recommended that the filter is changed regularly. Not all nebulizers have filters so check your manufacturer instructions. But if your nebulizer does have a filter, it should be changed regularly to assure you extend the life of your nebulizer and that the person using it, is breathing in clean air.

Purchase filters that are made for your nebulizer. Look at the owner's manual to find out which ones you need for your specific machine. Buy more than a few, and change it even more often than expected if the filter appears dirty.

Medication Care for the Nebulizer

- Make sure the medication for the nebulizer has not expired
- Check that the medication is not cloudy, or that the ampule the medicine is in, is not damaged

- Keep the medication in a cool place, and only refrigerate when there are instructions to do so
- Wash, dry, and store the equipment according to manufacturer instructions
- Have an extra tubing and cup available

(Information obtained from JustNebulizers.com)

Nebulizer machines do not last forever, especially if they are used 3-4 x/day. Consider getting a new nebulizer every few years to get the best efficiency from it. My patient, Gigi, was complaining that she felt her nebulizer was not working very well. I noticed that her machine must have been at least 5 years old. It was taking 30 minutes to get one nebulizer treatment done. I ordered her a new machine, and she said, after one treatment, that she was breathing better and the treatments took half the time.

How to Use/ How to take care of oxygen equipment (Oxygen Concentrators/ Nasal Cannula)

People who suffer from COPD (Chronic Obstructive Pulmonary Disease) and other types of lung disease, benefit greatly from the use of oxygen. There are other conditions that may require supplemental oxygen in order for the person to stay more active, and have a clearer mind. These conditions are pulmonary hypertension, bronchiectasis, lung cancer, and black lung (pneumoconiosis).

An oxygen concentrator is a free-standing machine that draws the oxygen from the other gases in room air. According to the American Thoracic Society (ATS), a nasal cannula connected to the oxygen concentrator delivers 90 to 95% pure oxygen directly to your lungs.

Oxygen therapy will need to be ordered by your HCP. A person needs oxygen when their arterial blood gas is below 88. An oximeter is a device you can put on a finger and can tell you what your oxygen is, but is not as accurate as of the arterial blood gas test. It is a good diagnostic marker for determining if oxygen delivery is working. You can order an oximeter online, but be sure to go over with your provider what are the acceptable readings, and keep a record in your daily logbook.

When you turn on the concentrator, watch where the little ball goes to on the gauge (called a flow meter). The ball will sit on a line between two numbers. If the number below it is 2, and the one above is 4, then the oxygen is set at 3 liters/minute. Make sure not to increase the oxygen flow rate without your provider's orders. Some medical problems, like COPD, only allows oxygen levels up to 3 or even lower, to prevent delivery of too much oxygen.

Oxygen Concentrator Care

- Always check your manufactures instructions for care
- Clean the outside once a week with a damp cloth and mild soap, never use spray cleaner
- Check to see if you have filters on the outside of the machine; if so, remove them from the oxygen concentrator and run them under warm water /mild soap detergent
- Check that the filter is not damaged in any way, and if it is frayed, or ripped, it will need to be replaced
- The tubing connects to the concentrator on one end and the nasal cannula on the other end. It does not need to be cleaned, but replaced every 6 to 12 months, according to the ATS.

Humification for the Concentrator

Humidifiers do not always come with your concentrator. It is used for comfort, especially in the winter months when the air is dry. The oxygen user may complain of dry throat, and nose bleeds, especially when using the oxygen all of the time. You can check with the vendor what humidification bottle they can send you to connect to your concentrator. All you do is fill it with distilled water. When you turn on the oxygen, you will see bubbling in the bottle. Every now and then, unscrew it from the concentrator to run warm water in the bottle to clean it.

Portable Oxygen

The oxygen that is portable is in oxygen tanks of either compressed or liquid oxygen. You will get pure oxygen from them. The tanks can be ordered by your provider to give you more mobility to get up and about. It is important to know how long the tank lasts so you can bring a spare with you, so you do not run out. Be sure to keep your spare tanks in a rack sitting upright at all times.

Let's go over the parts of a portable oxygen tank: First is the cart that holds the oxygen tank. Above the tank is a circular dial called the regulator. The regulator tells you how much oxygen is in the tank by watching the dial move from FULL on the right to EMPTY on the left. The flow meter looks different than the one on the concentrator. It is attached on the other end of the regulator and is a dial you turn to the ordered number. On the side of the flow meter is where you would attach the nasal cannula.

How to assemble a new portable cylinder

- First place the patient on another source of oxygen
- Turn off the flow meter from the old cylinder
- Turn the top fitting on the cylinder yoke clockwise with a cylinder wrench
- (that came with the oxygen) to close the cylinder
- Loosen and disconnect the regulator from the empty cylinder
- Discard the plastic gasket
- Remove the plastic band from the full e-cylinder

- Flush the cylinder by quickly opening and closing the top fitting on the yoke
- Take the plastic gasket which is on the new cylinder and attach it to the regulator
- Attach and tighten the regulator to the yoke of the new cylinder using the cylinder wrench
- Turn on the flow meter to the prescribed flow.
- Listen for the sound of air, which is the oxygen flowing
- Reattach the patient with the cannula to the new cylinder

The Inogen One is a portable oxygen concentrator you can use for long periods of time without the worry of running out of oxygen. It is lighter and smaller than an oxygen tank, allowing easy mobility and independence.

Nasal Cannula Care

- Clean the cannula once a week and as needed
- Wash the cannula in soapy water and rinse it with 10 parts water to one part vinegar.
- Rinse thoroughly with hot water and hang to dry

How to apply a nasal cannula tubing:

- Make sure the cannula is clean
- Put the cannula with prongs facing towards you, curving downward into your nostrils
- Loop the tubing around the ears
- Gently pull up on the small connector to keep the tubing under your chin

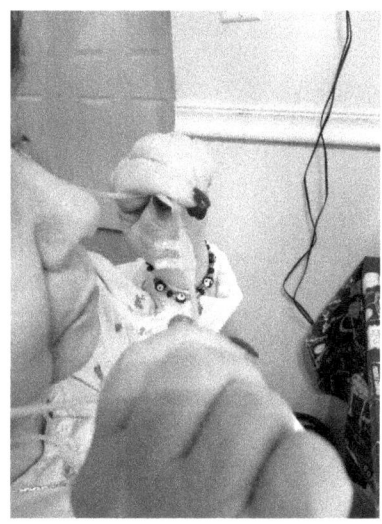 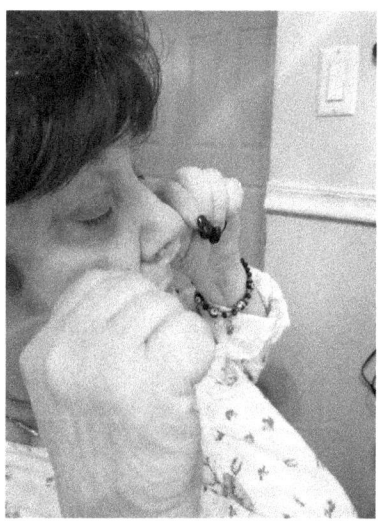 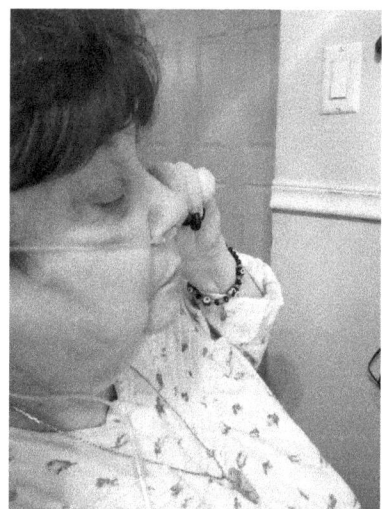

If you notice some redness behind the ears from the cannula tubing, you can either wrap the tubing with soft gauze where it falls behind the ear or take a small hair clip and pull the tubing up over the ears to the back of the head. Clip the two sides of the tubing together with the clip. Make sure the hair clip is not pinching the tubing. If the nasal passages get dry from the cannula, get some over-the-counter nasal saline. It is easy to use by squirting a small amount up into each nostril.

If the nasal cannula is not working out, you could get an adult face mask from your vendor. It is more constricting, but it works better for some people.

How to Use/ care for your/BIPAP, CPAP machine

- Always keep your owner's manual for troubleshooting
- Remove the water reservoir for humidification, and fill it daily with distilled water to the fill line
- Pop it back in the back of the machine
- Insert the electrical cord in the back of the machine and plug into the wall
- Insert the tubing to the humidifier opening on the machine

- The SD card is in the back of the machine and records your compliance with night use, so your health provider to see it when you go to the medical office so, leave it in place
- Connect the mask to the tubing
- When ready to go to bed, put the mask on, then turn on the machine

Cleaning your CPAP machine

- It is important to keep your CPAP clean, as it becomes a reservoir of mold, and bacteria that can make you sick
- Wipe the case with a soft wet cloth
- In the back of the machine are the filters:
- Remove the filter weekly and clean it with soap and water
- Remove the disposable filter and replace it every 30 days
- The hose should be disconnected and hung to remove excess water every day (you can put it over the shower curtain pole)
- Using a long brush, you can clean the hose with soap and water
- The CPAP bacteria filter needs to be changed every 6 months

There is a kit called Control II solution you can purchase from various vendors. Check out SoClean2 machine on YouTube that can clean your mask and water reservoir from your CPAP machine using ozone. It takes a total of 2 hours to work. There is also Lumin - so check them out. They thoroughly clean your equipment and will save you time.

What is an Incentive Spirometer?

It is a device you hold in your hand that may be ordered by your HCP to help with lung function. The device encourages you to take slow, deep breaths. Conditions that warrant its use are: pulmonary disease (COPD), asthma, sickle cell disease, emphysema or asthma.

Safety tips while on oxygen therapy

- Stay at least 8 to 10 feet away from open flames- including candles and stoves. Electric razors have been known to cause a spark, so do not wear oxygen while using an electric razor.
- Do not smoke or have others smoke around you.
- Avoid using aerosol spray products as they are combustible and cause a fire.
- Do not allow any flammable liquids to get onto your clothing
- Keep your oxygen concentrator in an open area, not a closet. This area is confined and can cause heat build-up
- Be sure to alert your power company you are on oxygen, so they put you first in line for power restoration. Also, consider negotiating a lower rate, so your concentrator is more affordable.
- Oxygen hoses now come in green color so you can see them on the floor. Be careful not to trip on the hose. (There are devices online that actually reel up the oxygen like a vacuum electric cord, that you can take with you room by room.)
- Make sure you put a sign stating there is oxygen in the home, on the main door of the house/apartment.

Check out the website "Do more with Oxygen" for downloadable self-help booklets, blogs, and equipment.

Check out under Durable Medical Equipment about the care and use of the nebulizer, oxygen concentrator, suction machine, and CPAP machines.

Safe Storage and Disposal of Medications

Your mother is living in your home with your adult children. There may be drug seekers and you are unaware. It is very important to keep all medications that contain any form of narcotic in a safe place.

Once the medication is no longer needed, it is important to dispose of it- either bring to your nearest police station or pack the medication (uncrushed) in a zip lock bag with kitty litter or coffee grounds, then throw it away. Take medicine out of the original container and remove the label with the person's name, address and prescription number on it, or use a black magic marker to blacken out the information.

Another product called Deterra can be purchased online. It is a package that deactivates the medication. Just pour the medications into the package and add warm water. Wait 30 minutes then discard the package into the trash.

You can contact your local city or county government's household trash and recycling service to see if your community has a medicine take-back program. If you have questions about discarding your medicine, call 1-888-INFO-FDA (1-888463-6332) or check out FDA.gov.

Saving Energy When You Have a Chronic Condition

Having a chronic condition such as Chronic Obstructive Pulmonary Disease (COPD), Congestive Heart Failure (CHF), or any other long-term condition can zap your energy to live your life. But if you can learn some tips to save your energy, you can be less tired and still have the quality of life you are striving for. Going through a cardiac or pulmonary rehabilitation program can make you breathe easier. Also, physical therapy and occupational therapy can equip you with devices for reaching, walking and improving strength so you can continue to be independent.

I have a patient who cleans her bathroom from her wheelchair on Monday, her refrigerator on Tuesday, washes clothes on Wednesday....you get the idea.

- To conserve energy, first make a list of what you do every day and put all the tasks together by location
- Do the chores in one part of your home around the same time of day
- Do errands or chores when you have the most energy
- Make sure to plan rest periods
- Sit down as often as you can when you get dressed, do chores, or cook
- Having a 4-wheel rolling walker with a basket allows you to carry items from place to place, such as spices in the kitchen or laundry to the machine
- You can push items in boxes instead of lifting them; consider putting them on some kind of wheels

- Move items you use the most on the lower shelves in your closets at shoulder or waist level so you can get to them easier
- Use the long-handled grabbers to get things off the higher shelves

I was in a department store, where I noticed a woman and her elderly mother (probably in her late 80's), who was walking with a quad cane. For an hour while I was there, I noticed her everywhere I was: looking at blouses, jewelry, cooking items. Her daughter had a cart and was buying items while mom kept up. I noticed her looking in a mirror smoothing her hair, holding up a blouse to her chest to see how it would look on her.

She must have walked two miles in that store! I stopped the daughter and asked her how often her mother goes out shopping with her. She said at least 3 days a week. Tomorrow is the grocery store where she holds onto the cart and pushes it around the store. What a great way to get exercise! If you don't use it, you lose it!

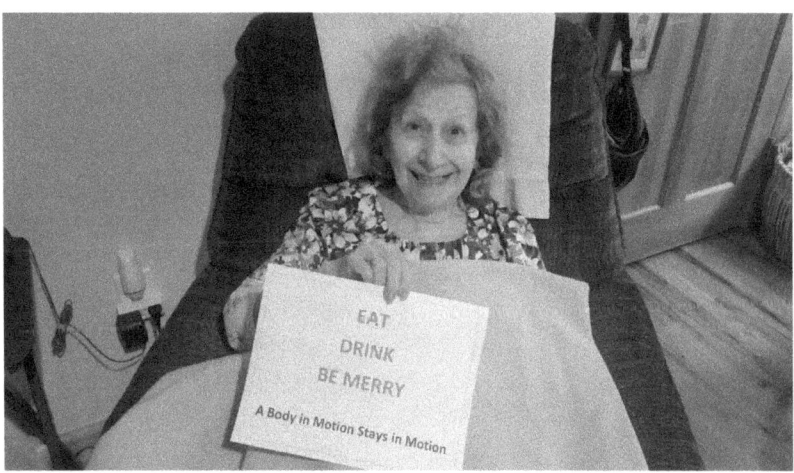

I also have emphasized that the person being cared for should be an active participant in their care. For instance, after having her hair washed, hand her the comb and have her raise her arms up as much as possible to comb the front and back of her head. Hand her the washcloth with soap on it and have her wash her thighs, and if she can bend down a little, have her wash her legs, etc. We need to keep moving in order for our muscles to continue to function well and to prevent weakness from lack of use.

In addition, everyone should be doing some degree of exercise every day. Put on the music and have the aide or family member direct the person- clap your hands, raise your arms up and down x 10, lift one leg and then the other x 10. Start at the top of the body and work your way down. Every joint should be moved as best as you can, and with a few repetitions. This is called Active Range of Motion.

Passive Range of Motion is when the person cannot move their extremities on their own, and you need to do it for them. During a bath is a great time for the person to have joints moved. As the aide washes the person either in bed or on a tub seat, she could move from first the head, gently turning the head left to right, then chin to chest, then back; then moving to the hands, fingers, and wrists, etc. By performing this on a daily basis, and more often with undergarment changes, joint contractures and joint stiffening can be avoided.

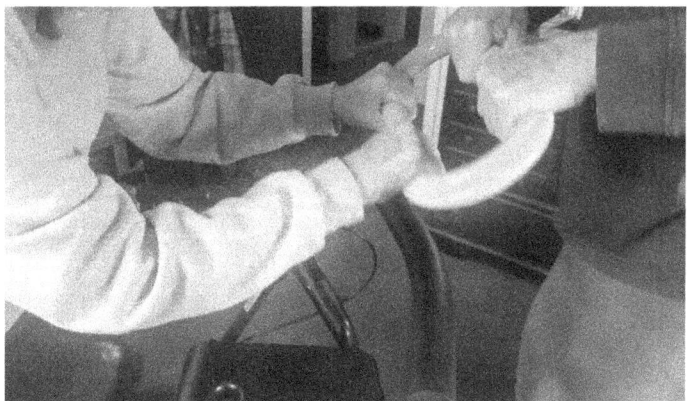
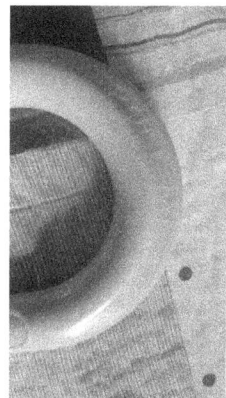

The Pull Me Up Device was one way to reduce straining of the back and other injuries that the caregiver could experience during a transfer. There are all shapes and sizes available on line.

Social Isolation in the Older Adult

Social isolation is becoming prevalent among this generation of Baby Boomers since many are divorced, widowed, their children have moved to areas that are cheaper to live and the Baby Boomer is aging in one place. Their parents from the earlier generation remained married until death and the family remained nearby.

Social isolation is defined as the absence of social interactions, contacts and relationships that include friends and family. Take my mother- in -law, for example. She was a very social being and she traveled on an RV with her husband living in more than 3 states in their lifetime. They made many friends of whom they played cards, camped and shared many happy memories.

Her husband died and so did 95% of their friends. Steve's mom is very hard of hearing and is isolated socially because she cannot carry on a conversation with friends when in a group. She would say that when she goes to church, she could not hear the sermon. She would get daily texts and calls from her children, but it is not the same. When her husband was alive, at least she knew he was in the other room and she felt his presence.

The longer a person is isolated, the more health risks he/she will endure and the mortality rate will increase. Eating alone can lead to weight loss. The person can become depressed, weak and be at risk of falling. Steve's mom did have a strong faith in God which kept her mentally strong and grounded. During the Covid 19 Pandemic, I was called by Mom to come get her. She was hoping to move up with us sooner but then realized that she may get detained in Florida as the country was shutting down.

I did take a plane from NYC to Florida only to find myself on a 747 with 15 people. I spent 8 days at her home, cleaning, packing, visiting her friends and driving back to CT with her. She was so relieved to be with her family again.

Moving to an assisted living facility and having your own room, meals prepared, and regular activities provided may still cause people to feel lonely and isolated. The person has to be willing to engage with others in order to find those that are like-minded. The remedy is to continue to make new contacts and keep the old, if possible. Be involved in your church/synagogue, meet your neighbor and reach out to your family to let them know how you feel.

Here are some books that can help you deal with isolation: *How to Overcome Loneliness and the Fear of being alone while Learning to Love Yourself* by Janett Menzel.

Emotional First Aid by Guy Winch P.H.D. This book is written for anyone who is looking for more resilience, building of self-esteem and to let go of hurts and hang-ups that are holding you back.

Social Workers- What can they do for you?

Social workers are Master's level helpers who observe, listen and counsel from a biopsychosocial perspective. They consider an individual or family's social environment, culture, personal psychology, family history of illness, etc.

Why might I need a social worker to help care for my loved one?

When your family member has behavioral issues due to dementia, Alzheimer's disease, bereavement, depression, anxiety, etc., a social worker can help to diagnose the problem and make treatment recommendations. For example, Joan is the daughter of an elderly married couple who lives out of state. She is an only child. Joan's parents are becoming progressively unable to take care of their ADL's (activities of daily living). Joan knows that her mom has a history of hoarding behavior, obsessive-compulsive disorder (OCD) and anger issues. Her dad has always depended on his wife to take of him, but she is declining and can no longer manage her spouse's care.

What does a social worker do to help?

In the example above, the social worker might make a home visit to assess issues that are making the situation problematic. The social worker is one-part detective, one-part healer, and one-part connector.

(Resources: Check out the National Association of Social Workers)

Spirituality - Finding your peace, and how faith gives you hope

There comes a time when we may become more reflective of our lives and what may be waiting for us after we die. We may find ourselves embracing religious beliefs more and more. Beit Judaism, Christianity, or any other religion, we become more in-tune to our religious upbringing and what our beliefs are. We become closer to what we were taught when we were younger and what we feel is right.

Some things we cannot change, but our attitude, we can. Taking time to sit on a rock and listen to a stream, or watching the clouds move across the sky, or just imagining being someplace beautiful. These tasks can bring more peace to your life. Consider yoga, meditation, listening to scripture as ways to help with daily coping. There is a new app called "Hallow" that has a daily devotion.

As part of my spiritual journey, I have been a faith community nurse for the last 7 years for my local church. Congregations from all religions need advocacy from the health professionals. We have formed a Health Council incorporating all health professionals, not just nurses. The mission of the council is to provide spiritual, educational and emotional care. We strive to advocate to alleviate suffering, facilitate healing and optimize health and abilities to our parishioners, their families and our surrounding community.

How to use/ Care for your Portable Suction Machine

- Always tell the person what you are about to do, give reassurance
- Place the suction machine on a sturdy surface and plug it into an electrical outlet
- Most suction machines work on an internal battery should the power go off, but works better when plugged in
- Make sure there is some water in the bottom of the collection container
- Wash your hands thoroughly with warm water and soap for 20 seconds, dry hands well
- Obtain:
    - disposable gloves
    - sterile suction attachment
    - tubing to the suction machine
    - a large cup of distilled water
- Connect one end of the tubing to the collection container and the other end to the suction catheter
- Place the cup with distilled water close to the bedside
- Check the tubes to make sure that they are all secured before turning on the suction machine
- Turn the ON button on the machine
- Adjust the pressure of the suction if desired
- Place the patient in a comfortable position sitting up, or on her side with head up to 30 degrees
- Don your gloves, and remove the wrapper from the suction catheter

- Have the patient open her mouth and push the suction catheter slowly towards the back of the throat. If the patient gags, pull back on the catheter and stop suctioning.
- Suction for small intervals
- Suction the distilled water in the cup into the catheter between each suction
- When you are done, turn off the suction machine
- Empty the collection container in the bathroom sink or toilet, rinse and fill it with a small amount of water for next time
- Never let the fluids collect higher than the line on the collection container
- Never suction for more than 15 seconds, as it reduces the person's air intake
- ALWAYS talk to the person during any procedure

How to take care of your suction machine

- Always keep your owner's manual for reference
- Wipe the machine with a moist cloth, then dry
- Keep it on a surface and away from heat
- Check the filter on the bottom of the machine (white knob) and inspect for dust
- If there is dust, remove it or consider replacing the filter
- Clean the collection container with warm soapy water after each use; you can put a small amount of mouthwash in it.
- Make sure the suction is working by turning on the machine and placing a finger over the opening on the machine where the tubing attaches. You will feel your finger being sucked in
- If there is no suction, check if there are cracks in the collection container
- If so, you will need to replace it by calling the vendor

Telehealth

Telehealth is a virtual program that HCPs use to evaluate, diagnose and treat patients using technology. Use of a video conference and a smartphone a patient and clinician can communicate without an in-person visit. The program works well for minor and non-urgent problems. During the Covid 19 pandemic, telehealth was the lifeline for so many people. It has become reimbursable by most insurances.

Telehealth is also used in a large extent for mental health counseling. There is something comforting and easy about sitting on your couch and having a session with a counselor in the comfort of your own home.

There are three categories to classify Telehealth: remote patient monitoring, store-and-forward and interactive telemedicine. Remote patient monitoring allows people with chronic medical problems to be monitored in their own homes such as blood pressure or blood sugar monitoring. Lab results are shared between two clinicians in the store-and-forward process. The third tool is actual fact-to-face real time sessions between a patient and the clinician. This is a great way to keep people out of the emergency and, hopefully out of the hospital.

Tornado Safety Tips

Gather the following items, so you are prepared:

- Flashlight and extra batteries
- Battery-operated radio and extra batteries
- First Aid kit
- Emergency food and water
- Non-electric can opener
- Essential medicines
- Checkbook, cash, credit cards, ATM cards
- Designate a friend or family member to be available to check on your elderly parent

Transportation

When you are no longer able to drive, there are ways to get around. It is not easy to be told you can no longer drive as you do not pass your driver's test. Uber or Lyft has become our newest "taxi" service.

Also, check with your local Office for the Aging as you can get registered for TRIPS which are buses that can come get you, even if you are in a motorized wheelchair. You need to register with TRIPS in order to get this service. Also, you need to have an appointment for the bus to pick you up. They have a ramp in the back of the bus that transports you onto the bus without getting out of your wheelchair. If you work with a house calls company, they may have contacts for you, such as retired people who want to work per diem, and are willing to drive you places. After all, they could become your personal chauffeur!

Another great driving service is GoGoGrandparent. Go to https://get.gogograndparent.com or call 855-9535-1490. This service is available in all 50 states, Canada and Australia. They are a service that sets up drivers with people who need transportation, groceries, pharmacy delivery, meals, home chores and more. Of course, there is DoorDash and Instacart for delivery services.

"Upsizing" Your Home

So many older people live in the same home they raised their children in living in only 4 of the 9 rooms. High ranches were the homes built in the 1950s, which were fine when you had a young family. But having to go up a set of stairs or down as soon as you enter the home as an older person, made their home a "prison." The people I would see would stay upstairs and never leave the home because of the stairs.

I have imagined that someday, if I live long enough, I would consider renting out bedrooms and would share the kitchen, hire a housekeeper and live-in aide, and as I aged, I would have companionship, independence in a home, someone to cook for my roommates and myself. All we would need is a traveling clinician such as myself, to take care of the medical needs and monitor for any signs of problems.

Maybe two good friends could live together but even better if separated by an apartment door, so as to maintain privacy. One such situation I experienced was with one of my patients named Mary and her best friend from 4 the grade, June, who had this arrangement.

Both families bought and refurbished apartments that were next to each other, connected by a door. They each had live-in aide, had most meals together and went to adult programs for dementia during the day. The bittersweet part is that they remembered each other well, but became very forgetful about many other things and people. June died and Mary would ask where she is all the time. The children were able to downsize their homes, give them companionship, and they got an investment for their future. More people should consider this idea.

I also had a family of 4 people: divorced male, and his three female cousins who were widowed. They all moved in together and pooled their pensions, social security checks, and resources to take care of each other. They lived like this for over 20 years, and just recently Eddie, the caregiver with myasthenia gravis could no longer take care of Eleanor, the remaining resident when they both went into a nursing home. I took care of Eleanor, who was bedridden for over 7 years.

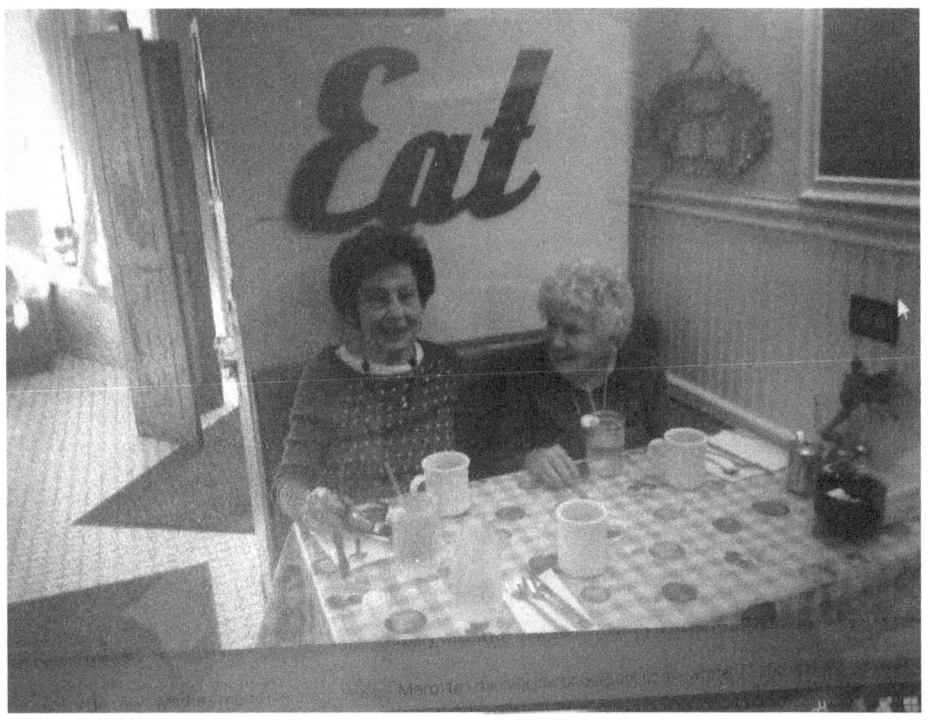

Many of the people from the 50's era, did not think about getting rid of unused memorabilia over the years. We, the children did not help as we left our Barbie dolls in the attic, old clothes, boxes of pictures never digitalized, and some of our furniture from college. Mom and Dad's home became our place to leave stuff behind as we went on to live our lives. Not to mention graduation pictures on the wall of their children who are now 30 years older.

When my dad moved, all 7 of us children had to claim our belongings or say goodbye to them because they would have been thrown out. This was the impedance for us to declutter the home and simplify his life. I took my high school yearbook, some love letters, and my nursing cap.

At this time in my life, I am finding it necessary to purge every year by getting rid of old papers, furniture, and items I have not used or worn over the last year. While the things are in good shape, it is time to sell them on eBay or Craig's list, give them away to someone you know or just leave them out on the curb for someone of interest to pick up. Somehow you get the feeling of peace and control. Besides, I want to live on a boat, and there is nowhere to hang a picture, so we need to keep it simple and practical.

I recently read an article by Joshua Becker, author and editor of "Becoming Minimalist" who talked about shedding yesterday for a brighter today. The article talks about how our "home is a launching pad from which we live our lives in the world." We know the longer we live in a home, the more it collects objects from our past. We keep things because they remind us of good times or we think we might need them again. But we need to realize that life has changed.

When we get rid of excess possessions it is about releasing an older version of ourselves. And this is where we struggle. Decluttering our things from the past can almost feel like we are betraying the past or have lost appreciation. The article goes on to say that "by decluttering possessions from previous seasons of life, you don't diminish that season. We do just the opposite. You honor it by fully embracing the new you that was formed out of it." The acknowledgement that those items served their purpose in shaping us, and we also must give ourselves permission to move forward.

So, back to Mom who is in that house from 1955 and she is now 90. What to do! Check out my video on my YouTube channel, Caregiver Success, called "Do you need to Declutter? with Jean Marie Herron.

If you look online, there are services out there to help with downsizing.

One such company is called Home Again Transitions. This company has professionals that help sort belongings, disposal or "repurposing" of items you will not be taking, packing, and unpacking you in your new home. They help you save time, energy and money while reducing stress.

They service most of New York and Westchester but do have a large network across the country of companies that do the same thing. It is a tough conversation to say to your mom or dad about making a change in the home. Check out the website to get tips about how to start the conversation. "Everyone has a scary room, closet or drawer," the website says.

If this company is not in your area, you can call them, and they will help you network with people in your community. Call David and Debbie Feldman at 914-734-9187 and check out www.homeagainny.com. By going to their website, you can get monthly emails of tidbits to help with the transition. You can also go to nasmm.org and put in the locator your zip code to help find a transitions coordinator in your area.

There are also great books out there to help you get equipped with the information and tactics to help with change. *Guiding Our Parents in the Right Direction (Practical Advice about Seniors Moving from the Home They Love)* by Bruce Nemovitz, and *Moving in the Right Direction,* same author.

Another consideration is to stay in the same home but make changes so that your mother can "age in place." Many of our parents who bought homes in the '50s have stayed in them for more than 60 years. They have no mortgage but pay taxes and utilities. Sometimes selling the home to move into a senior housing may cost more than staying in one place. If the home has been kept up throughout the years, renovations to age in place could be done sparing little expense.

Living in a ranch is the best idea yet. Aging in Place is a concept where kitchen counters could be lowered, rails placed in the hallways, taking out the tub and making a walk-in stall for a shower. Doorways can be widened for wheelchair access.

You Can Stop Smoking

Any habit is hard to break. Sometimes we just reach a breaking point. I remember my friend, who was a heavy cigarette smoker, who had an epiphany as he was putting the key in the lock of his front door. He noticed how yellow his door was and he knew what this was from: all the cigarettes he had smoked over the years. Well, that was the breaking point. He emptied his pockets of cigarettes, went through his cabinets and hiding places and threw them out. He actually quit on the spot. This is not easy to do. He then had his entire home re-painted, especially the front door.

The reasons to quit smoking

One of my patients moved in with her daughter in a smoke-free home. She had her own apartment attached to the home, but you could smell cigarettes when walking in the home. She was an 84-year-old woman who smoked since she was 16. She had her first smoke before breakfast and the last one before bed. She would rather smoke than eat, so she lost weight. She had emphysema and was short of breath with little exertion. Her quality of life was not very good.

One day, the aide found her unable to speak and she was hospitalized with a mild stroke. Her daughter told her she could not smoke in the home any longer. While in the hospital, she could not smoke and was given nicotine patches. By the time she came home, she was no longer a smoker.

So, why should you quit smoking? Did you know that smoking remains the leading cause of preventable death and disease in the U.S. and is known to kill more than 480,000 Americans each year? We all know that smoking is related to the possibility of lung cancer. Adults exposed to second-hand smoke are also at risk of lung cancer, heart disease, stroke, leukemia, and lymphoma. In addition, a cigarette contains 69 cancer-causing agents and 7,000 toxic substances. Smoking slows down healing because of the reduction of oxygen circulating through the bloodstream which helps with repair.

It is when you start thinking of quitting; you are already taking the first step. First, consider reducing how many cigarettes you have a day. Try to stretch one box of cigarettes to cover a longer period of time. Open a small bank account to deposit the money you would spend on the extra boxes of cigarettes. You could plan what you would want to spend the money on as a treat: a trip, clothes, etc.

As far as helping someone cut down on smoking, spend more time with stimulation such as playing cards, singing to music, looking at old photos, to reduce interest in that cigarette.

Some tips on how to quit smoking easier:

- Make one list of why you smoke and one list of why you should quit; take time to compare them
- Keep this list and look at it from time to time when you have the urge to smoke
- Set a target date to quit
- Throw out old ashtrays and lighters
- Tell all your friends and family that you have set a date to quit so they can be there to support you and keep you accountable
- On the day you quit, clean all your clothes, burn a scented candle, and consider getting your teeth cleaned
- Have your carpeting and furniture steam cleaned
- Have healthy snacks like celery, or fruit to help with oral satisfaction

- Whenever you feel a craving to smoke, take deep breaths in and out slowly. Stress is a trigger to smoke, and deep breathing helps with relaxation and calm
- Drink plenty of water, as water helps with nicotine detox. Water will be filling so you do not eat more, and it loosens mucus so you can clear your lungs
- Meditation helps with envisioning good thoughts and mental pictures to help curb actions and reduce cravings
- Try to reduce caffeine intake since nicotine makes it less potent, and when you quit smoking, caffeine is more of a stimulant. Caffeine increases the heart rate and can lead to insomnia.
- A stress ball can help you find something to do with your hands instead of holding a cigarette.
- Take up new interests like cooking or painting to take your mind off of smoking
- Healthy exercise to replace an unhealthy exercise of smoking will make you feel better due to the release of good-feeling dopamine.

If you have smoked for a long time, consider seeing your HCP for Wellbutrin and a nicotine patch program. You would start the Wellbutrin at the time of the quit date. It is a mild antidepressant that can make you feel better since you would be "losing your friend, the cigarette." The nicotine patch is started at a dose based on how many cigarettes you smoke a day and is reduced every few weeks as you reduce your craving to smoke.

You may not be very successful with quitting the first time, but keep trying!! And remember, you are never too old to quit!

(http://www.cdc.gov/tobacco//data_statistics/fact_sheets/)

Quitline Services:

1-800-QUIT-NOW (1-800-784-8669) free phone support service that can help people who want to stop smoking or using tobacco.

When you call this number, callers are routed to their state quit lines who will then offer you different types of services:

- Free support, advice, and counseling from experienced coaches
- A personalized quit plan
- Practical information on how to quit, including ways to cope with nicotine withdrawal
- The latest information about stop- smoking medications
- Free or discounted medications
- Referrals to other resources

Mailed self-help materials: (https://www.cdc.gov/tobacco/data-statistics/factsheets/cessation/quitting/index.htm)

Winter Safety Tips

I arrived to visit 86-year-old Gigi and found her in a very cold home, wearing a wool hat, 3 layers of clothing and was under covers with an electric blanket. She told me that one of her pipes broke due to the cold and that the plumbers are coming today to fix it. Gigi lives alone in a big old house and tends to roost in her bedroom, migrating only to the kitchen and bathroom as needed. I waited for the plumbers to come as I could not leave her alone until the heat came on. I warned her about the use of an electric blanket as it could cause burns on the skin or a fire. She said she would remove it once the heat is on.

Winters conditions are very dangerous, especially for the older person.

Here are some tips from the Office of Fire & Emergency Services:
Before a winter storm strikes:

- Listen to the local emergency alert system stations updates
- Get a snow removal service in place
- Use rock salt, kitty litter or sand on walkways
- Winterize your home: double pane windows, rugs on floors, bumpers against leaky doors
- Have your water boiler and heating system maintained
- Check smoke detectors
- Have some type of safe emergency heating equipment available such as a safe free-standing heater
- Fill up the tub with water, if there is a chance for a winter freeze

Winter Health Hazards

Frostbite

A severe reaction to cold exposure that can be permanently damaging. Symptoms include a loss of feeling and a white or pale appearance in fingers, toes, nose and ear lobes.

Hypothermia

The body core temperature drops below normal. Symptoms include shivering, slow speech, memory lapses, and drowsiness.

What should you do?

If these conditions are suspected, slowly warm the person with blankets, offer something warm to drink like tea or broth. DO NOT give the person anything that will make them sleep and no alcohol — **call 911**.

Section II

MEDICAL CONDITIONS OF THE OLDER ADULT

Anemia

Anemia is defined as a condition where either the red blood cells are lower than normal, or they do not include enough hemoglobin (Hgb). Hemoglobin carries oxygen through our blood to tissues and organs. A symptom of anemia is fatigue and with long-term anemia, there could be damage to the brain, heart and other body organs.

What causes anemia?

Blood loss is the most common cause of anemia and is called iron deficiency anemia. Cancer, surgery, bleeding in the urinary or digestive tracts and trauma are causes of blood loss anemia.

The second cause is a lack of production of red blood cells. This condition is either inherited or acquired. Causes can be from chronic disease, diet or hormones that prevent a person's body from creating red blood cells. Also, factors that destroy red blood cells are at a high rate needs to be evaluated. If someone has an enlarged diseased spleen, more blood cells are made than are needed. In this situation, the person needs to give blood to reduce the number. An inherited condition would be sickle cell anemia.

Risk factors for anemia include low iron, low vitamin or mineral diet, long-term illness (cancer, diabetes, HIV, heart failure and thyroid disease). If the mean corpuscular volume (MCV) is high, it can mean a vitamin B12 or folate is deficient. If the MCV is low, consider serum iron depletion and it needs replacement. A simple blood test called a Complete Blood Count (CBC with differential, vitamin B12, folic acid and serum iron) can help determine what type of anemia you have.

Arthritis- osteoarthritis or rheumatoid

One day I had such pain in the joint of my right index finger. Boy, that smarts! Now I have a deformity at the tip of my finger, and I know what it feels like to have arthritic pain. Arthritis is inflammation of one or more of your joints causing pain and stiffness that worsens with age. There are two types of arthritis that are the most common- osteoarthritis and rheumatoid arthritis.

Osteoarthritis is caused when the cartilage that covers the ends of bones begins to break down causing a "bone on bone" condition; whereas, rheumatoid arthritis (RA) is an autoimmune condition (a condition where the body's immune system attacks itself) and involves the lining of the joints. With rheumatoid arthritis, the lining called the synovium, becomes swollen and inflamed. Soon the cartilage and bone can be destroyed.

Osteoarthritis causes a restriction in movement, such as walking, getting out of a chair or just using your hands to stir your coffee. This condition happens over the course of years or can happen sooner if you had surgery on a joint, such as a hip or knee; or due to an infection of a bone. Both of these conditions can change your ability to carry out daily activities.

Who is at risk for arthritis?

- Look at family history- your genetic makeup can trigger this condition like it did in your family member.
- Age- the older we get, the more we are at risk for getting arthritis.
- Sex- females are more likely to develop rheumatoid arthritis, while men are more likely to develop gouty arthritis, another type.

- History of a joint injury- those that injured a joint from sports, a car accident or surgery, are at risk of developing arthritis.
- Obesity- Being overweight, causes excess weight on the joints that support you (hips, knees, and ankles) leading to arthritis.

What are some things you can do if you suffer from arthritis?

Acetaminophen (Tylenol) is typically the first line of treatment for mild to moderate pain caused by osteoarthritis. If the pain is more severe, acetaminophen could be added to an opioid, such as tramadol.

Exercise

- Apply moist heat to joints for 20 minutes before exercise
- With osteoarthritis, no pain no gain. You need to keep moving because if you stay in that chair, you just get stiffer and stiffer. The pain in the joints do not improve with lack of movement. Get up every hour and walk around, making sure to move arms and legs, etc. Exercise strengthens muscles around your joints, gives you more energy, and improves your balance.
- Keep the impact low and slow
- Apply ice to joints for 20 minutes after exercise
- You may notice some pain after exercise, but if you are sore 2 hours later, then you exercised too strenuously
- Do not overdo!
- Use good posture
- Consider rehabilitation with a physical therapist or occupational therapist for a home exercise program.
- Also watch YouTube for chair exercises

RA is first diagnosed by seeing a rheumatologist. He/she will determine what medications you could take to prevent further breakdown of the synovium while treating the pain. (Mayo Clinic site 2019)

Aspiration- How to Prevent it

Dysphagia is a medical term used to describe swallowing difficulties. Aspiration is when a person starts to cough or choke while eating or drinking causing food or liquids to enter the airway and lungs instead of the stomach. Symptoms of aspiration are a runny nose, tears, coughing, throat clearing, or gurgle, and wet voice when speaking.

A modified swallow study will show the action of the fluid going down the esophagus and will tell you if the person may need a feeding tube. The tube provides nutrition without chronic and repeated episodes of pneumonia from aspiration.

You can examine the person's swallowing by watching the "Adam's apple" move up and then down. It also helps when someone "holds" the food in the mouth, to remind her /him actually to swallow while you touch the throat to remind him. Go slow when feeding and avoid having the person talk while there is food in the mouth.

Liquids can be thickened by using such agents as Simply Thick (gel format) or powders to make a nectar or honey consistency. The liquid should "glop" off the spoon, not "drip," indicating that it is thick enough to ingest. If there is still some coughing during drinking, then just thicken the liquid even more. Using thin straws, the ones for stirring, are better for drinking than the thicker ones since they reduce the amount of fluid going down throat at one time.

Simply Thick can be purchased online as a premade solution in a jug or easy mix packets. I like this product because all you need is a fork to whip up the liquid and you can make a whole pitcher. It does not settle or get gloppy as other products do. Arrow root powder can be purchased in the grocery

ASPIRATION- HOW TO PREVENT IT

store and can be used to thicken liquids and soups, etc. This is a cheaper version and works like Simply Thick.

See the next picture of a cup with a cut in the side. This U-shaped opening allows for a person to drink without having to tip the head back fully so to allow liquids to go down the esophagus instead of the windpipe (trachea).

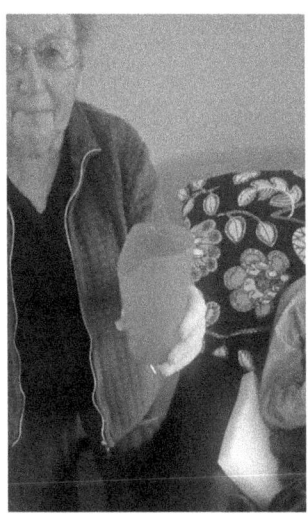

Tips when eating or drinking:

1. Sit upright when eating, and make sure the head and chin are in a 90-degree angle. (Try putting a rolled-up towel behind the neck to push the head forward)
2. Stay upright for 20-30 minutes after a meal
3. Feed liquids with a spoon
4. Between meals, make sure the mouth is clear and clean
5. You can give a few spoonsful of water (not thickened) even if she coughs a bit.
6. Liquids should be thickened (as above)
7. Foods should be soft and moist (see below)
8. Soups should be thickened

Using the Blender

It's time to be creative with food. Puréeing a beef stew tastes just as good as chewing on meat and carrots. Shakes with berries, thickened oatmeal with bran and banana, or chocolate pudding with ice cream for a treat, work great for those with dysphagia. The idea is to make the meal interesting but also safe. As a person loses weight, their dentures do not fit the same and would need to be adjusted.

Atrial Fibrillation (AF)- what exactly is this?

Atrial Fibrillation is an abnormal heart rhythm that feels like the heart is fluttering. It can be a constant feeling, or can happen periodically. The upper chamber of the heart, called the atrium, is where the abnormal beat comes from. Sometimes there are no symptoms but it can be heard with a stethoscope and confirmed with an EKG, a complete history, thyroid blood work, and CBC as well as echocardiogram. Sometimes, there are complaints of dizziness, fainting, shortness of breath, or even, chest pain. As we age, our risk of developing AF increases.

What happens is the 2 top chambers of the heart, called the "atria" (atrium is singular) quivers or fibrillates instead of contracting, avoiding a sufficient amount of blood filled with oxygen to enter into the lower chambers of the heart called the "ventricles." This blood sitting in the atria can pool and clump together. This is how clots are formed. If a clot is there, it can break off and travel to the brain leading to a stroke.

Depending on which part of the brain is injured, it will determine what the disability may be for a person. The most common occurrence is becoming paralyzed or very weak on the entire side of the body. Some people have trouble with word finding, swallowing, or walking. Having a stroke can lead to more events of stroke. But it can be easily diagnosed as a possibility by having regular medical exams.

This disease can lead to an increased risk of heart disease, and dementia. People with hypertension (HTN) or those with diseases of heart valves, heart enlargement, and coronary artery disease are the most common risk factors for AF. This condition increases with age, especially over the age of 80. Smoking increases the risk of AF 1.4 times more than that of non-smokers.

AF is treated with medications called "beta blockers" to slow the heart rate to a normal range. A cardiologist is a specialist to determine if other methods are needed to reduce the heart rate. A low-dose aspirin or anti-clotting medications such as Coumadin may be ordered.

AF can be caused by having diseased heart valves or not. Non-valvular AF has a chance of causing a stroke 5x/ more than if the valve was diseased. There are other medications such as Plavix or Eliquis that do not require blood monitoring like Coumadin does. Your cardiologist will help determine what your best treatment be.

KardiaMobile Main unit is a portable device that can capture a medical-grade EKG in 30 seconds with the results appearing on your smart phone. Simply place your two fingers on each pad. The EKG can then be shared with your cardiologist or HCP.

Cancer in the Older Adult

As we age, the risk of cancer increases significantly. Cancer at an early stage is usually operable and would be beneficial to do if it can improve the person's quality of life. I visited one woman who did not tell anyone in her family that she had drainage from her left nipple for over a year. When I examined her breast, she had a folded maxi pad in her bra that was saturated with drainage. She had a large visible mass on the breast. She stated that she was 87 years old and knows that this is breast cancer but does not have any pain and does not want surgery. She was willing to have a DNR in place so no heroic measures were taken.

On the other hand, my father had prostate cancer when he was 75. He did not have it removed and had seeds implanted and had radiation. He lived to 94 without recurrence of cancer or problems from prostate cancer. He did not suffer from urinary incontinence either. A total prostatectomy has more chance of causing incontinence. It is always good to weigh risks and benefits before deciding whether or how to treat any cancer. Because prostate cancer is genetically predisposed, my brothers need to have their prostates checked as they age.

There are some cancer screenings that are discontinued once the person reaches a certain age. According to the USPSTF, this preventive list is changed based on statistics. You can google the Medicare Learning Network. For information about cancer care, go to www.cancer.org.

Congestive Heart Failure (CHF)

I never liked this term. I felt like people would think that their heart has stopped working or has failed them. What heart failure means is that the heart muscle that pumps the oxygen and blood to your organs of the body is not doing a great job. Therefore, you can develop some symptoms that can reduce your quality of life.

CHF is one of the top medical diagnoses that lead to hospitalization for people over 65. If you follow good healthy habits and take your medications, you can prevent hospitalization. The medical conditions that put you at risk for developing CHF are coronary heart disease, heart attack, high blood pressure, and diabetes. Behaviors that can increase your risk of developing CHF is smoking, eating foods high in salt and fat, little physical activity and being overweight.

An echocardiogram will determine the movement of the heart and the size of your 4 heart chambers. The left ventricle, which is the lower right chamber of the heart, gets enlarged called "hypertrophy," and causes the pumping action, called the ejection fraction (EF) to be low. According to the American Heart Association, the EF should be between 55-70% for a normal heart.

You may be given the following medications:

Beta-blockers

They slow heart rate, decrease blood pressure and improve your condition
Example: (Metoprolol)

Angiotensin-converting enzyme inhibitors (ACEIs)

They reduce the heart's workload, lower blood pressure, and reduce leg swelling. (example: Lisinopril) Beta-blockers and ACEIs are important medications to take every day if prescribed because they will reduce hospitalization.

Angiotensin II receptor blockers (ARBs) work like ACEIs

You may be given this medication over an ACEI; sometimes people complain of a cough from Lisinopril or other ACEIs. (example: Diovan)

Diuretics

(also called water pills) like Lasix, help with leg swelling and remove extra fluid from the circulation.

Potassium supplements

Potassium can be lost when on a diuretic. Therefore, these supplements may be added to your medication list.

Aspirin or other blood thinners

These medications can be used to prevent heart attack or stroke.
    Do not take any vitamins, over-the-counter medicine, or herbal products without talking with your HCP or pharmacist first; and also, do not take Advil or Motrin, or Aleve without checking with your HCP as it can cause worsening of CHF.

How do you avoid exacerbations?

- Keeping a weight log by weighing the person the same time every day, and recording it
- Ask your HCP if you need to limit the amount of liquids a day
- Sleep on one to two pillows at night to make breathing easier
- Avoid high sodium foods (check out low sodium diet under "Eating Healthy for Older Adults"), this includes fast foods, restaurant foods, boxed foods
- Eat fresh: fruits, vegetables, lean meats
- Avoid using the saltshaker
- Take your medications as prescribed and do not run out of them
- Report to your HCP if your abdomen is distended (right-sided failure is when the fluids back up from the heart on the right side affecting the liver and abdomen).
- Elevate your feet above the heart to prevent edema (swelling). You should be able to see your toes in front of you.
- Avoid getting sick from colds and flu. Get a flu shot every year, and check with your HCP if you need to get a pneumococcal vaccine
- If you smoke, ask your HCP how to quit
- Lose weight if you are overweight
- Be sure to keep your medical appointments

Some of the warning signs that you are having an exacerbation of CHF:

- Edema (swelling of the legs and feet)
- You have trouble lying flat in the bed because it is hard to breathe
- You may notice increased distention of the abdomen
- You may be "winded" when walking up the stairs

Call your HCP **now** if:

- You have new or increased shortness of breath
- You have a sudden weight gain, such as 3 pounds or more in 2 to 3 days
- You have increased swelling in your legs, ankles, and feet
- You are suddenly so tired or weak that you cannot do your usual activities

Call **911** if:

- You have severe trouble breathing
- You cough up pink, foamy mucus
- You have a new irregular heartbeat

Constipation

Constipation is defined as having fewer than two bowel movements per week, and it is hard to pass stool. What may be considered a normal bowel pattern for one person may be different for another. Constipation can exhibit pain in the rectum and cramping. No one likes to be constipated, especially if you are bedbound, and may not be able to verbalize how you feel. If your mother has a good appetite, then she should have a bowel movement every day or every other day.

When a person is sedentary and does not drink enough liquids throughout the day, and does not have much fiber in their diet, they will certainly become constipated. If the person becomes dehydrated from medications such as diuretics (Lasix), anticholinergics (Ditropan), calcium channel blockers, anti-inflammatory agents such as Motrin and Advil, narcotics for pain (e.g. Tylenol with codeine), and antacids that contain aluminum, constipation can occur.

The following medical conditions can contribute to constipation as well: diabetes, stroke, Parkinson's disease, depression, dementia, and other types of illnesses that cause salt and water metabolism problems.

My strong recommendation is to hang a calendar in the bathroom or near the bed and mark off the date, time the bowel movement occurred and if the bowel movement is small, medium, or large. The calendar becomes a quick visual of the week.

Coffee and stewed prunes have a laxative effect for many people. Foods high in fiber are: bran, beans (like lentil, navy beans) split pea, broccoli, sweet potatoes, and nuts. All vegetables have some degree of fiber.

If the person is on a diuretic like Lasix, she may have harder stools which are more difficult to pass and can also lead to hemorrhoids (indicated by rectal pain, and scant bleeding seen on the stool). If the person finds themselves bearing down too much, more serious problems can occur such as a rectal fissure, which is a tear in the rectal wall, or fainting on the toilet.

The condition where the person faints on the toilet is called the Valsalva maneuver. It is where the person forcefully breathes out with mouth closed, causing a change in heart rate and blood pressure. People have been known to fall off the toilet sustaining injuries. If constipation becomes a chronic problem, consider going to a gastroenterologist.

Bowel Regime

First drink plenty of fluids, enough, so urine is light yellow or clear, like water. Make sure to check with your HCP if you have kidney, heart or liver disease, as limitation of fluids may be warranted. Include high-fiber foods as mentioned above. Get at least 30 minutes of exercise a day such as walking around your home or outside. Consider using a small stool in front of the toilet to place your feet. This position helps flex the hips and places the pelvis in a squatting position.

Some older people just need a stool softener, such as docusate sodium (generic for Colace). A great product that I recommend is polyethylene glycol (MiraLAX). It has no taste so can be easily added to any drink, and does not get sludgy. Since most people have difficulty taking the full capful in 8 ounces of liquid, I recommend splitting up the dose- 1/2 cap in 4 oz of morning coffee, for instance, and the other 1/2 in 4 oz of juice at lunchtime. For most sedentary patients, they do well with taking the stool softener and MiraLAX daily. Citrucel or Metamucil in small doses to start can help.

If constipation continues, consider Dulcolax suppositories which stimulate the bowel below, and Milk of Magnesia 2 tablespoons orally at the same time. An enema such as the Fleets over the counter is only temporary help and should not be used as a regular measure, as the muscles in the colon can become weakened and dependent on the enema for bowel movements. Probiotics are known to help with a healthy gut, and so, can improve constipation. Check out www.nutrametrix.com/mobilemedicalhealth for probiotics.

Constipation versus Diarrhea

The reason for keeping a bowel calendar is so you can watch the story unravel as to whether there is indeed constipation. If the calendar shows no BM for 4-5 days, and diarrhea as loose, watery stools, there may be a large piece of stool blocking the lower colon leading to this oozing of brown liquid around it. I would do a rectal exam to see if the stool can be felt, and as graphic as this sounds, actually remove the stool digitally. This stool is considered impacted. Sometimes the patient then has an evacuation of a large amount of stool. The emergency room staff frowns on stool removal.

I sometimes order a flat plate x-ray of the abdomen in the home, and if there is "large amounts of stool throughout the colon but no distention or severe impaction," I have the caregiver give one bottle of citrate of magnesia at night, and call me the next day to tell me of the results.

Deep Vein Thrombosis (DVT) -What is it and how to you prevent it?

DVT is a blood clot that develops in the vein of one of your legs. For clotting to occur, the vein was either damaged or the blood flow had slowed down. The veins involved are either superficial (on the surface of the leg) or deep (deep in the leg). Most of the time the DVT is in the deeper veins. A DVT that occurs below the knee is not as dangerous as one that is behind or above the knee. A DVT above the knee has a bigger risk of breaking away from the vein and traveling to the lungs, which can be life-threatening.

Situations that increase the risk for DVT:

- Being over the age of 40
- Being obese
- Active cancer and its treatments, which can cause the blood to clot more easily
- Dehydration
- History of clotting
- Immobility (being bedridden, not walking, or paralyzed)
- Hormone therapy (used for menopausal women)
- Surgery lasting more than 30 minutes, especially if it is on the legs
- Long-distance travel with sitting too long

Signs and Symptoms of DVT:

- Swelling of the leg or around a vein in the leg
- Pain or tenderness felt when standing or walking

- Warmth and redness of the leg
- The risk of a DVT is the traveling of a clot to the lung called Pulmonary Embolism (PE). PE can actually cause sudden death.

Symptoms of PE that require a 911 call:

- Difficulty breathing
- Heart rate is elevated
- Chest pain
- Coughing up blood
- Very low blood pressure
- Dizziness or fainting

How is a DVT diagnosed?

- You will need a full medical history and physical exam by your HCP
- The leg will need an ultrasound to look for the clot
- Venography (x-ray that shows the blood flow with the use of dye)
- Studies to check for clotting problems in your blood

Treatment for DVT:

The most common treatment is taking an anticoagulant, or blood thinner such as Warfarin (Coumadin) every day. Blood work called PT/INR would need to be checked every 2 weeks or so, to check that the medication is in a therapeutic range. There is a device called Coaguchek that allows the person to take their blood test at home, then call the HCP with the results to determine how much Coumadin to take daily.

Blood thinners can be dangerous medications. If a person has a falling history, an injury to the head can cause extensive bleeding and could lead to death. Also, these medications cause slow healing since clotting is part of the healing process. So, if a wound is involved, it will not heal very quickly.

Compression stockings are used to relieve pain and swelling, and to prevent a condition called "post-thrombotic syndrome." These stockings, also called TEDs, are tight elastic tubes that start at the foot and go up to the knee; and sometimes, up to mid-thigh. The compression is at 100% at the foot, 70% at the calf, and 40% at the thigh. These stockings come with a hole where the toes are so you can check the person's circulation while wearing them.

Many of my patients hated them because they are so difficult to get on and off. There is a product called Tubi grip that is elasticized tubing that comes on a roll. You can cut them and discard them if they get soiled. They are easy to put on because they do not have a fitted foot portion. You can buy them online. Another company called Medi makes a variety of products, which includes colored stockings, so they look less conspicuous. Check out www.mediusa.com.

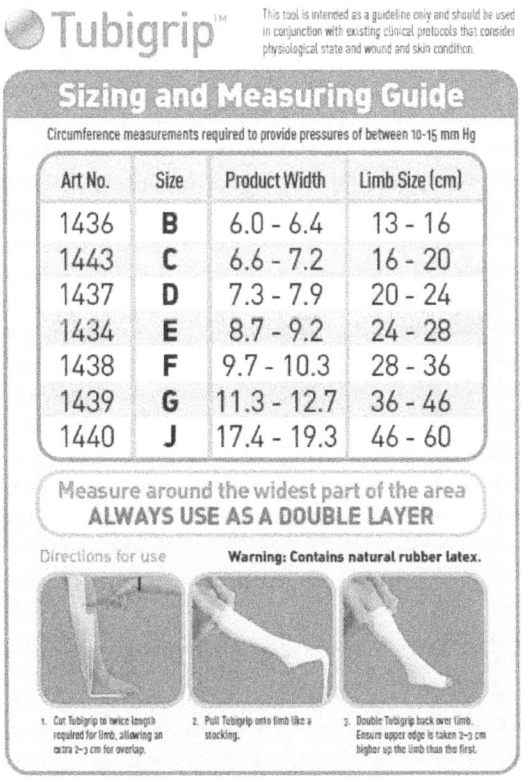

Compression stockings are taken off at night and are easier to apply before stepping out of bed in the morning since the swelling in the legs and feet are at their lowest point. There are many variations on line of a product for easy application of TED stockings. Doff N' Donner is such a product. It is a donning device for all types of compression socks and stockings. It allows independence or easy application for the caregiver.

Most people with DVT are advised to place a cushion under their feet while resting or sleeping so that the feet are raised higher than the hips. This helps to reduce the pressure in the veins of the calves.

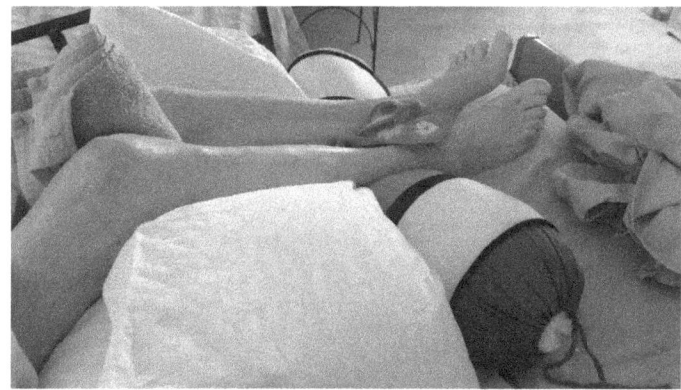

(See the section about the application of compression stockings, ACE wraps, and Tubigrip).

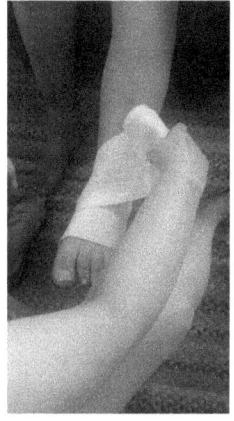
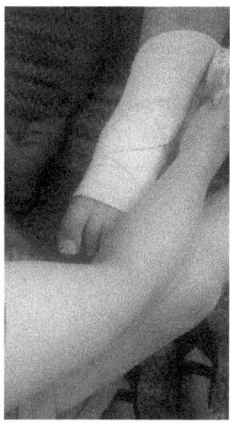
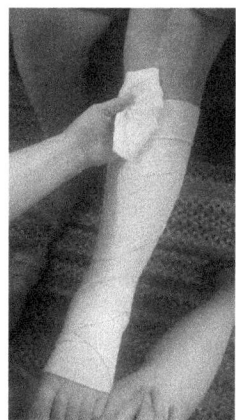

General Preventive Advice for those at high risk of DVT:

- Exercise the legs regularly- and if you can walk, do so for 30 minutes daily
- Maintain a weight appropriate for your height
- Avoid sitting or lying in bed for long periods of time without moving the legs
- Wear loose-fitting clothes to prevent constriction
- Keep legs uncrossed
- Keep hydrated

Venous Ulcers

The valve in a vein act as a door, so as the blood flows up the vein in the leg, the valve prevents the blood from flowing back down. A DVT can damage the valve causing blood to pool in the lower leg. This is called post-thrombotic syndrome, and causes chronic leg pain, swelling, discoloration and leg sores, called venous ulcers. The leg becomes discolored, the circulation becomes impaired, and sores called venous ulcers can develop.

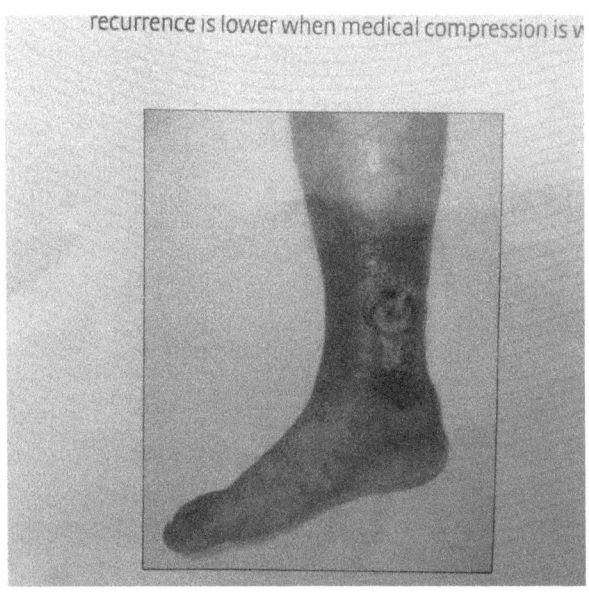

Dehydration- What should you watch for?

Did you know that our body consists of at least 60% water? Dehydration occurs when a loss of fluids exceeds fluid intake. Our bodies are constantly shifting with fluid moving in and fluid moving out. Even a minor change in fluid concentration can result in dehydration. This includes wounds with excessive discharge, weeping of fluids from the skin due to cellulitis, or diarrhea to name a few. Fever, vomiting, excessive sweating and medications such as Lasix can also cause fluid loss. Older people tend to drink less, so to avoid going to the bathroom; hence, dehydration ensues.

Symptoms of dehydration:

- Bad breath- lack of saliva causes bacterial overgrowth
- Fainting
- Sunken eyes
- Rapid heartbeat
- Rapid breathing
- Very dry skin
- Sleepiness, lack of energy, confusion or irritability
- Fatigue (a build-up of lactic acid can occur with fluid loss decreasing glucose production)
- Dark yellow urine-when we are hydrated our urine is clear with a tinge of yellow
- Headache-salts such as potassium sodium are lost when we lose fluids. Loss of water in the brain tissues causes the brain to shrink away from

the skull. When this happens, the pain receptors in our head become sensitive and can cause headaches.
- Crying without tears and a dry tongue and mucosa inside the mouth
- Loss of the skin elasticity-the skin should snap back when pinched. When dehydrated, the skin remains elevated for a moment then returns to normal
- Call your HCP if you suspect mild or moderate dehydration.

How do you treat dehydration?

Dehydration must be treated by replenishing the fluids in the body. Drink clear fluids (which are any fluid that when held up to the light is clear), is the person is having diarrhea: apple juice, chicken broth, water, seltzer, tea, Gatorade. Stopping water pills temporarily, such as Lasix and hydrochlorothiazide (HCTZ) may be necessary. Drink enough fluids so that the urine becomes pale and more frequent. Avoid caffeine, fatty foods, alcohol, and tobacco.

Weigh the person every day, if she can stand, and record the weight to see if she is gaining. If she has a temperature of 99.4 F orally or higher, keep a record of it every 4 hours and call the HCP if the oral temperature is over 100.4F.

Severe dehydration shows a rapid, weak pulse, cold hands, and feet, loss of ability to sweat, blue lips, confusion and difficult to awaken, with barely any urination. This situation requires hospitalization right away.

Liquids come in all forms

Water is not very tasty, and as we get older, our taste buds change, and flavors are not the same. There are all sorts of supplements out there that can provide a caloric intake of 350 calories in a can or bottle. You can find them in 6 packs in most pharmacies and grocery stores. When the person has a poor appetite, two cans a day of a supplement, such as Ensure, can allow 700 calories out of 1500 calories that is needed/day. Glucerna is a good supplement for the diabetic since it is low in sugar.

    Jell-O works great, ice cream with or without sugar, soups, tea, broth, juices or making your own smoothies filled with berries, juice and crushed ice all put together in a blender. Anything that is liquid at room temperature is a liquid, so be creative!

The Aging Brain

As the brain ages, it gets smaller in size and reduced weight. Mental processing can be delayed. However, dementia is NOT a normal part of aging.

Here are some warning signs of dementia:

- Memory loss that disrupts daily life
- Challenges in planning or solving problems
- Difficulty completing familiar tasks
- Confusion with time and space
- Trouble understanding visual images, like pictures
- New problems expressing words and speech
- Misplacing things and losing the ability to retrace steps
- Decreased or poor judgment
- Withdrawal from work or social activities
- Changes in mood and personality

(Alzheimer's News. Know the 10 Signs: Early Detection Matters. E-newsletter. Alz Assn. 2009. Last assessed online Nov 19, 2012.) Http://www.alz.org/national/documents/checklist_10signs.pf

When the person with dementia comes out of a hospital or nursing home, he may be belligerent and confused for a few days. Most clinicians try to keep people with dementia out of a facility because when they are taken out of familiar surroundings, their behavior can change.

Types of Dementia

Dementia can be a slow or rapid process, where the person loses the ability to remember names, events, day-to-day activities, and worst of all, their loved ones caring for them. Sometimes, a person can get more than one type of dementia. Based on the location in the brain that is affected, speech, personality, memory, ability to care for themselves, called ADLs "Activities of Daily Living," comprehension, depression, and anxiety can occur.

Here are some types of dementia:

- Alzheimer's dementia
- Frontotemporal dementia
- Lewy Body dementia
- Mixed dementia (Alzheimer's & Vascular)
- Parkinson's disease
- Vascular dementia
- Alcohol related dementia

(Landau SM, Harvey D et al. Comparing predictors of conversion and decline in mil cognitive impairment. *Neurology.* 2010 Jul 20; 753):230-8.)

A neurological exam by a neurologist along with a CAT Scan of the brain are both necessary to determine a person's neurological status. A Mini-Mental State Exam (MMSE), clock drawing, and PHQ-9 are tools used to score the extent of dementia, and the later, for depression.

(See a sample of the MMSE and PHQ-9 depression screen in the Glossary)

In addition, blood work to check Vitamin D, thyroid, vitamins B12, folic acid, VDRL (syphilis test), CBC for evaluation of anemia, and infection, and a urinalysis to rule out a urinary tract infection. The person needs to be given a diagnosis of dementia in order to start treating to slow down the progression of the disease.

A medication called Aricept, a cholinergic which is known to slow down or hinder the advancement of dementia, may be started. The drug is started at 5 mg at night for a few weeks then increased to 10 mg. It is known to cause diarrhea. Also, Aricept counteracts some medications used for overactive bladder, which are anticholinergic such as Detrol. Namenda (memantine) is a medication also used for Alzheimer's disease and works by decreasing abnormal activity in the brain by a different mechanism than Aricept.

Antidepressants are frequently started for the older adult as serotonin, a hormone in the brain, depletes with age, causing symptoms of depression. Usually, the MMSE is repeated in 6 months to check for a change in the score after trying any of the above medications.

Also, the PHQ-9 depression screen scores for depression. PHQ-9 stands for Patient Health Questionnaire which scores each of the 9 DSM-IV criteria as "0" (not at all) to "3" (nearly every day). It has a maximum score of 27. Elevated scores strongly correlate with a major depression diagnosis.

Delirium versus Dementia

Delirium is a sudden change in mental status which can occur within hours or a few days. The person could be sleeping all the time, not eating, has smelly urine (which could mean a urinary tract infection) and cough (which could mean pneumonia). Dehydration can change behavior causing her to be more aggressive or having hallucinations. Some medications could contribute to delirium: Benadryl, Thorazine, and Parkinson's disease medications; and opioids (OxyContin, Hydrocodone, Fentanyl, Tramadol, etc.)

The difference between delirium and dementia is that delirium is usually reversible, where dementia is not. (Mayo Clinic Nov 2011).

Here is a mnemonic to help you to think delirium:
D- Drugs (anticholinergics, opioids, alcohol w/d, dopaminergics
E- Electrolytes (Na, Ca, BUN, glucose)
L- Lack of Drugs (pain, alcohol use, Rx meds)
I- Infection (UTI, aspiration pneumonia)
R- Reduced Sensory Input (restraint, hearing, vision)
I- Intracranial (rare) meds, seizure, stroke
U- Urinary Retention, fecal impaction, meds
M- Myocardial, PE, MI, CHF

It is important to seek medical attention if you suspect delirium. A careful history and exam are needed by your HCP to perform a cognitive and neurological exam: the MMSE and head-to-toe assessment; labs to include CBC, complete metabolic panel, thyroid test, Vitamin B12, folate, urinalysis, blood test on medications that require levels, like digoxin or Keppra. Also, have the lungs checked, and it is good to check oxygen levels, maybe a chest x-ray and ekg. The staff and family should assure a safe environment for the patient, avoid using any type of restraints or other methods of immobility.

Medications such as Risperidone, Seroquel, and Zyprexa may be ordered to help with the treatment for delirium.

(Wilber ST Onndrejka JE. Altered Mental Status and Delirium. Emergency Med Clin North Am. 2016 Aug:34 (3): 649-65.)

My friend, Jynx took care of her husband, Axel with Alzheimer's dementia for over 9 years. She would tell me how he loved to fix cars, and build things. He was worked as an Automotive Engineer, Manager of Product Analysis and Expert Witness for Mercedes-Benz NA Corporate Office. He was highly intelligent and witty.

She said she would start seeing small changes. As I was visiting Jynx, she showed me the garage where everything was always meticulous and organized. He would spend hours there with his son, Jamie, building furniture and tinkering with cars. He started buying multiple saws, and other equipment of which he did not need. The garage became very disorganized, and eventually, he stopped going in it, as he lost interest due to his advancing dementia.

When I took care of him, I could see how hard it was for her. She was realistic about what was going to happen based on the progression of the disease but watched him become more dependent on her. In his last 3 years, Axel was no longer mobile, and she hired a live-in aide for $1000/week. She went through a large portion of their retirement. She said no one seemed to understand that after all that time caring for him and then he died, that she was "suddenly no longer employed." She says she was saying goodbye to different parts of him every day. (see Ambiguous Loss at the end of the book)

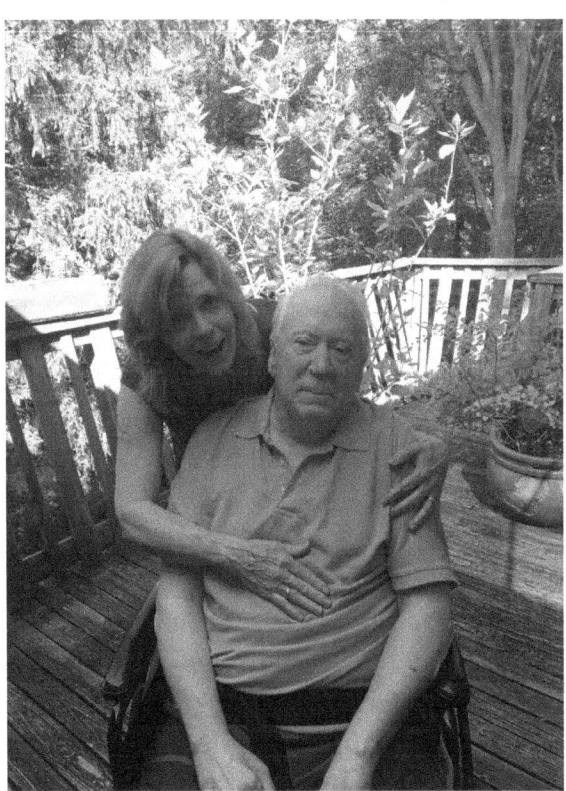

Jynx always treated Axel with respect. She remembered how cool he was, and how much fun they had together. She spoke to him all the time. She was patient and encouraged him to be independent, to be part of his own care, and make decisions for as long as he could. She cooked healthy meals and cut up his food carefully. She would lie with him in his hospital bed at night until he fell asleep because he suffered from sundowning. I marveled at her dedication and love for Axel.

Jynx found this poem and passed it on to me:

An Alzheimer's Poem

Do not ask me to remember
Don't try to make me understand.
Let me rest and know you're with me.
Kiss my cheek and hold my hand.
I'm confused beyond your concept.
I am sad and sick and lost.
All I know is that I need you to be
With me at all cost.
Do not lose your patience with me.
Do not scold or curse or cry.
I can't help the way I'm acting.
Can't be different though I try.
Just remember that I need you,
That the best of me is gone.
Please don't fail to stand beside me,
Love me 'til my life is gone.

By Owen Darnell

Diabetes Mellitus

Symptoms of Diabetes (high blood sugar):

- Frequent urination
- Sudden weight loss
- Wounds that will not heal
- Always tired
- Always thirsty
- Blurry vision
- Numb or tingling hands and feet
- Sexual problems

Symptoms of Hypoglycemia (low blood sugar)

- Shakiness
- Weakness
- Headache
- Dizzy or lightheadedness
- Sweating
- Irritability
- Hunger

What causes low blood sugar?

- Skipping a meal
- Not eating enough at a meal
- Taking too much insulin or diabetes medications
- Being more active during the day than usual

How do you know if your blood sugar is low?

Check with your HCP about what your blood sugar numbers are, and use a glucose monitoring device. If you feel your blood sugar dropping, treat the reaction right away.

What should you do?

- Take 2 tablespoons of raisins
- 4 oz of fruit juice
- 5 pieces of hard candy

Source: Adapted from the American Diabetes Association, (http://www.diabetes.org/type-2-diabetes/hypoglycemia.jsp)

As a diabetic, it is important to pick the low Glycemic Index (GI) foods and limit any in the higher GI ranges. Eating low GI foods can help prevent type 2 diabetes, heart disease, hypertension, and obesity. Protein-rich foods like fish, chicken, and meat contain no sugar so have no GI rating.

You have heard of hemoglobin A1c (HbA1c) but what is it exactly? On routine blood work, it is recommended by the American Diabetes Association to get a blood test to check your A1c to determine if you have developed diabetes. The A1c is a measure of your average blood sugar over a 3-month period. For a diabetic, the A1c should be less than 7.0%. If you have a strong family history of diabetes, it is important to have yearly monitoring of your fasting blood sugar and A1c. In addition, do all you can to keep healthy habits so as not to develop diabetes.

If you have heavy or chronic bleeding and your hemoglobin stores are low, your A1c will be falsely low. If you have iron deficiency anemia, your A1c result will be falsely high. Another important point is that labs have different values for A1c, so consider this when having labs interpreted. Everyone with diabetes should know what their A1c is.

For every point above 6%, add roughly 30.

If the A1c is 6 %- start at 126 as your average fasting blood sugar; if it is 7% add 30 to 126= 156, and so on.
A1c of 8= 183
A1c if 9= 212
A1c of 10= 240
A1c of 11= 269
A1c of 12= 298

Measuring fasting blood glucose:
If you have diabetes, it is important to get a glucose monitoring device. If you are not on insulin, you do not need to check your blood sugar every day. But when you do, the first time of the day to check is before breakfast; and 2 hours after any meal (post-prandial). The range should be between 80 and 130mg/dl before a meal and less than 180mg/dl 1-2 hours after the beginning of the meal. Make sure to talk with your HCP about your results.

To make sure your meter is giving accurate readings, you need to get a test solution from your pharmacy. This solution is used when you open a new bottle of test strips and to be checked on the first strip. There is a range on the back of the test strip bottle that the reading needs to be between. If it is not, it may be time to get a new meter.

Pre-diabetes or Syndrome X: I have a "little sugar."

Having pre-diabetes means your A1c is between 5.7-6.4% and a fasting blood glucose of 100 to 125, or glucose levels of 140 to 199 at the two-hour point of a glucose tolerance test (US News and World Report).

Once you have been told that your A1c is over 6.5% you are no longer in the Pre-diabetes stage and have diabetes. The important thing to know is that you can help reduce the chance of getting diabetes by losing weight, especially around the abdominal area, walk or exercise at least 1 and 1/2 hours a week, and eat lots of fruits and vegetables. For women, the waist circumference should be under 35 inches and for men, under 40 inches.

A microalbumin test is used to detect early signs of kidney damage in people who are at risk. Checking the urine for protein is important to have done at least yearly if you have type 1 diabetes, type 2 diabetes or high blood pressure. A urine microalbumin test is to detect small levels of a blood protein called albumin.

(Check out "Low Glycemic Foods" under Eating Well for Healthy Adults section)

Eating Right for Older Adults

Let's spend some time giving you a nutrition lesson about vitamins, minerals and how it affects blood work and how you feel.

We have all be told that having a lot of color on our plate means a nutritious meal and that eating fresh is best. Many frozen foods are flash frozen keeping in the nutrients of freshly picked produce making them a good alternative. Canned goods tend to have more sodium to keep in the freshness but are not good for those with HTN. Also, foods in a box where you "just add water or meat" have many preservatives, sodium, and chemicals. They may be cheaper to buy than fresh, but do not come without a price. That price, over time, can be a potential problem for your overall health and wellbeing.

My husband and I have a vegetable garden every year in Connecticut. I am a part of an organic waste program, where I collect leftovers, rinds, vegetable clippings, stale bread, etc. It becomes part of a large community compost. We plant organic seeds of tomatoes, kale, eggplant, 4 types of lettuce, cucumbers for pickling - dill and bread and butter, squash, and green beans. This year, we made sauces with Roma tomatoes, relish, bread and butter pickles, and dill pickles. Going out to the garden to pick a few eggplants and making dinner with them is truly farm to table.

As we get older, our metabolism slows down, and we do not need to eat as much as we did when we were younger. Keeping the weight off helps everything from heart, to joints.

For women 51 and older who are:

Sedentary: 1,600 calories a day

Moderately active: 1,800 calories a day
Active: 2,000 calories a day

For men 51 and older who are:

Sedentary: 2,000 calories a day
Moderately active: 2,200 to 2,400 calories a day
Active: 2,400 to 2,800 calories a day

People over 50 need more calcium, vitamin D, vitamin B12 and fiber to stay healthy. Eating a varied diet consisting of fruits, vegetables, fish, lean meats and dairy every day can ward off several diseases. Look for foods low in saturated and trans fats. Portion control is a must in order to prevent unwanted pounds.

Take a 9-inch plate. Now put a line down the center of the plate. On the left side of the plate can be all the vegetables you like. Now go to the right side of the plate and cut that section in half. Each of those areas should have a protein such as meat, no bigger than the palm of your hand, and the last section is for pasta or some starch. Do not pile the food high and do not go back for seconds. If you want to have pasta, measure one cup of cooked pasta, and that is your portion!

(Sources: U.S. Department of Health and Human Services, ADA Complete Food & Nutrition Guide).

Many grocery stores have online shopping where you can pick the foods and have them either held at the store for pick up or for delivery. When getting blood work done, it is good to know what foods to eat or avoid based on certain blood levels, such as calcium, protein, and vitamin D.

Let's talk about gout:

Gout is caused by the production of too much uric acid.

Foods that are high in purine break down into uric acid, and can trigger a gout attack. Ask a person who has had one of these attacks. They will tell you how painful it was.

Here are some foods or drinks to avoid or have in small amounts to reduce uric acid production:

(notice the list is almost the same for diverticulosis)

- Red meat
- Fish such as herring, sardines, carp, cod, haddock, salmon, trout, tuna, anchovies, shellfish
- Beer, alcoholic drinks, or beverages with high fruit sugar
- Caffeine- it is a diuretic which reduces the water in the body and allows the uric acid crystals to crystallize in the joints
- Organ meats (calf's liver, hearts, lungs, spleens of animals)
- Fried foods and pre-packaged foods that are fried in oil then baked
- Soda
- Rich sauces like Hollandaise, brown and white gravies

Diarrhea

If the person is having diarrhea, which means frequent bowel movements, mostly watery, and may be accompanied by a low-grade fever and vomiting, you may consider viral gastroenteritis as the problem. Usually, it starts with someone else being sick in the home, and within 48 hours you are feeling sick too.

Eating a bland diet without dairy is the first step to getting better. Dairy is hard for a sick gut to digest. Foods with spices and sauces are usually not desired when you have no appetite and irritates the gut. An old mnemonic is the BRAT diet: eat **B**ananas, **R**ice, **A**pple sauce, **T**ea, **T**oast; hard-boiled eggs, and jelly on your toast, not butter. Crackers are a good substitute for toast.

Diverticulosis

Diverticulosis is a condition that typically affects the lower portion of the large intestine or colon where sac-like out-pockets line the colon. When these pockets become inflamed, diverticulosis becomes diverticulitis.

The following foods can cause bloating, gas and irritation to the bowel including diarrhea, abdominal pain, and rectal bleeding.

Foods to avoid:

- Red meat
- Fatty foods
- Cruciferous vegetables: broccoli, brussels sprouts, cabbage, kale, cauliflower
- Raw vegetables
- Alcohol
- Soda
- Whole grains- wild rice, whole wheat, bran
- Spicy food

Avoiding seeds and nuts is no longer foods that need to be avoided as there is no real evidence that they cause flare-ups.

Protein:

The person is at risk for skin breakdowns as protein is needed to maintain good skin tissue and promote healing. When your body does not have enough of this essential element, it has a difficult time forming collagen- a necessary component needed for tissue healing. Albumin, which is protein, is measured in a blood test. If your loved one has a bed sore, protein can be lost up to 100 mg per day. This is because the wound can have fluid leakage of protein and electrolytes.

Therefore, offer foods that are high in protein: fish, all types of lentils, black beans, corn, Greek yogurt, quinoa, cottage cheese, almonds, pistachios, lean meats, soy, and peas. Dairy products such as 1 cup of milk have 8 grams of protein.

Here is how you figure out how much protein you need to take in per day:

Start with .36 grams/ pound; multiply your weight by .36; for example, if you weigh 100 lbs. multiply it by .36, and you need to take in 36 grams of protein /day. For the person who is a poor eater, supplements such as Ensure Plus or Glucerna (sugar-free) are great for protein supplementation. For example, one cup of Ensure Plus has 13 grams of protein and 350 calories. Glucerna has 10 grams of protein and is 200 calories/ one cup.

If a bedsore is involved, you will need a higher requirement of protein to help with wound healing. It is recommended to get 25-30 grams of protein with each meal, and 10-15 grams with each snack. Whey protein powder added with fruit and chipped ice in a blender is a great drink and treat, for someone who needs more protein supplementation. You can also purchase whey protein on www.nutrametrix.com/mobilemedicalhealth.

Vitamins and Minerals in Food

Iron:

Iron is an essential nutrient needed to make red blood cells and prevent anemia. Red blood cells are needed to move oxygen to every cell in your body. If you are told you have low serum iron (Fe), and your Hemoglobin (hgb), hematocrit (hct) and mean corpuscular volume (MCV) is low, then you have iron deficiency anemia.

When someone has iron deficiency, they look pale, are complaining of being tired all the time, have breathlessness or shortness of breath, dizziness, heart palpitations, pale gums and a shiny bald tongue called "glossitis."

Some other signs are dry skin, brittle nails, and crusting of the corners of the mouth, called "cheilitis." When you pull down on their lower eyelids, the conjunctivae are pale and not beefy red.

The foods that are high in iron are as follows:

- Lean beef
- Dark meat of the turkey
- Lentils, chickpeas and other types of legumes
- Pumpkin seeds- one ounce a day gives you one-quarter of your daily recommended consumption of iron. They also have trace minerals like K, zinc, and magnesium that are important for good heart health.
- Broccoli- one cup a day gives 10% of daily iron, and also contains vitamin C. Steam it in a pot with a steamer to keep in all the nutrients.
- Quinoa (whole grain) also contains magnesium, copper, and antioxidants. (Antioxidants guard the body cells from free radicals, which interfere with new cell growth preventing cancerous growth in the body.
- Spirulina - a blue or green colored-algae found in health food stores. It contains 50% of the daily iron. It can come in pill form.

Iron supplements such as Feosol and FeS04 can cause constipation and makes stools look black. Eating foods with iron can also change the color of the stool (BM). Pesto Bismol is also known to make stools black. Iron pills should not be taken together with calcium supplements or with dairy because foods such as cheese, and milk binds to the iron pill causing it to be inactive. You can take the iron supplement two hours after dairy, however.

So, eating a healthy diverse diet and supplementing when necessary for deficiencies can ward off all sorts of health problems.

- Dark chocolate- especially the one with cocoa gives you 10% of daily iron from one ounce.
- Spinach
- Tofu- used to substitute meat for the vegetarian. It comes in sausages and cubes.

Vitamin C

Vitamin C is important in improving anemia due to iron deficiency. This vitamin helps the body absorb the iron. It would be good to add 500mg a day to your daily intake.

Vitamin D most people seem to have a low vitamin D. It is known that the sun is the best source of vitamin D and is best absorbed through the skin. Due to sunscreens in makeup and the lack of sun exposure by many, vitamin D deficiency is quite common. Vitamin D has been linked to a multitude of diseases and conditions: depression, for one, heart disease, bones can lose strength causing unexplainable aches and pains, and weakened immune systems causing more susceptibility to upper respiratory infections.

If you get a diagnosis of kidney disease, keep track of your Vitamin D levels, as the kidneys are known to help with its production; but only if the kidneys are working well. Vitamin D helps your gut absorb calcium-rich foods which reduces weak bones and osteoporosis.

Foods that are high in vitamin D:

- Fresh fatty fish (salmons, sardines, mackerel, bluefish
- Cod liver oil- 1 Tablespoon a day, which not that great tasting and can be purchased in a gel capsule

- Eggs- 10% of the vitamin D needed a day; also contains choline needed for brain functioning to reduce memory loss, cognitive decline, learning disabilities, and nerve damage.
- Fortified milk
- Fortified orange juice- one cup has 20% of the daily recommended Vitamin D
- Greek yogurt- 1 six- ounce serving has 20% of the daily recommended Vitamin D
- Beef or calf liver- 3.5 oz contains 12% of the daily recommended vitamin D
- Fortified cereals- 3/4 cup contains 10% of the daily recommended vitamin D

Omega 3 is found in fish and can be taken in supplemental form: 2-3000IU/day. If they have a fishy after-taste, you can place them in the freezer and ingest them frozen.

Magnesium

Magnesium is mostly stored in the bones, and small amounts are in the muscles. Early signs of magnesium deficiency include fatigue, loss of appetite and vomiting. As the deficiency gets worse, muscle spasms and cramping can occur. Pumpkin seeds contain magnesium.

Fiber

There two types of fiber: insoluble and soluble. Insoluble fiber adds bulk and softness to the stool and passes through the digestive system quickly. This prevents constipation and long exposure to toxins. Soluble fiber is necessary to lower cholesterol absorption and blood glucose levels by delaying the absorption of sugar in the small intestine.

Why should we eat fiber?

There are many reasons. First, it provides a feeling of fullness which can help in weight control. Secondly, fiber adds bulk to our diets, and by doing so, it aids in digestion and elimination, keeping our bowel healthy.

How much fiber do you need in your daily diet?

The average American has only 10-15 grams of fiber a day, which is well below the recommended dietary guideline of 25 to 30 grams/day. Fiber should be increased slowly so as not to cause stomach upset.

Foods that contain fiber:

- Split pea, all beans like chickpeas and lentils, especially pinto beans and black beans
- Most vegetables: broccoli, avocado, artichokes
- Raspberries and blueberries, bananas (eat the fruit instead of drinking fruit juice)
- Pears with the skins
- Choose bran-based cereals or oatmeal for breakfast
- Add wheat germ to soups, salads
- Snack with healthy foods: popcorn, whole grain crackers, nuts
- Purchase bread with whole grain as the first ingredient you see

Potassium

The heart muscle needs this mineral to regulate blood pressure and make muscles contract. If potassium is too low in the blood, you may need to take a medication called Slow K or potassium 10 -20 equivalents per day by prescription.

Foods that are high in potassium:

- Bananas- one medium contains 400 mg of potassium
- Salmon- 3 oz has 500 mg of potassium

- Acorn squash- one cup is 650 mg of potassium
- Low-fat milk- has 400 mg of potassium in one cup
- Leafy greens: Bok choy, spinach, kale, Swiss chard

Calcium

When calcium is low in the blood, there is usually no symptoms; but there can be leg and muscle cramps, and changes in hair and skin texture. Calcium is a necessary mineral for strong bones, teeth, and a healthy heart. Everyone over 70 should take in at least 1,200 mg of calcium/day.

Foods high in calcium:

- Mostly dairy products; cheeses, soy milk, sour cream, yogurt; almond milk is loaded with 470 mg in one cup!
- Seeds- sesame, chia and sunflower seeds
- Dried figs
- Leafy green vegetables - kale
- Sardines, salmon, rainbow trout
- Spinach, broccoli rabe, kelp (farmed seaweed), okra, soybeans
- Beans- navy, capellini, and baby Lima beans
- Oranges
- Almonds

(All information was obtained from nutrition sites on the internet)

Low Glycemic Index Foods

The Glycemic Index (GI) of food measures how much a carbohydrate-containing food raises blood glucose levels. Glucose has a GI number of 100. It's rapidly broken down once consumed and sent to cells for energy, then stored in the muscles to be used later or converted into fat. High GI foods range in value from 70-100; medium GI foods range from 56-69; low GI foods range from 55 and below.

Many foods have high fructose corn syrup in them such as hot dogs and catsup. This ingredient is sometimes the first one listed on the label. High fructose corn syrup has a high GI score. Being the first on the nutrition label indicates that the food has the most quantity of this ingredient. As you go down the nutrition label, the ingredients in the food product become less. Sugary foods such as ice cream, candy, soft drinks need to be avoided by the diabetic since they have a high GI and raise the blood sugar.

Foods to choose:

- Bread: Ezekiel bread which had 6 different grains and low GI score; including pumpernickel bread.
- Leafy greens: (spinach, kale, lettuce, collard greens. GI score is less than 10.
- Vegetables that do not contain starch: broccoli, asparagus, green beans, peppers, and tomato. They have a GI score under 10.
- Oatmeal- GI score of 55
- Barley - GI score of 25
- Most fruits have low GI scores like berries, citrus, apples, and cherries. Watermelon, grapes, and figs are high. You can have them but in small amounts.
- Beans and legumes- have 1/2 cup at a time. They are all low in GI score.
- Plain yogurt with no added sugar
- Chia seeds, pumpkin, and flaxseed are good to snack on since they are low in GI.
- Pasta is low on the GI score when compared with bread and potatoes. The way to keep the GI score low is not to overcook it, "al dente" is great.
- Sweet potatoes- boiled have a lower GI score than when baked.

- All- bran, natural muesli, and granola are all good cereals to eat. Instant packets of cereals are high in GI score, so avoid them.
- Kefir- a grain that is a strong probiotic, rich in protein and Vitamin D.

Low Sodium Eating

Sodium is one of the chemical elements found in salt. Reducing high sodium foods is important for most of us. Americans eat way too much sodium. If your mother is on a high blood pressure pill, then sodium should already be reduced in the diet. Foods that are canned or in a box have more sodium than fresh or steamed foods. Eating foods that have added salt and sauces can increase your sodium intake.

It is important to look at food labels: The Daily Value for sodium is less than 2,300 mg/day. Next to every food package is the percentage of sodium in a measured serving. If the serving size says that it meets 19% of your daily intake, then there is still 80% left to find in foods during the day.

Here are some foods to avoid or limit because of high sodium content:

- Soy sauce
- Ham
- Salami
- Corned beef
- Hot dog
- Ramen noodles
- Sauerkraut
- Parmesan cheese
- Ketchup
- Shellfish
- Bacon
- Sardines

- Peanut butter
- Soups

Pick foods with labels that say "low sodium" which has 140mg of sodium or less per serving. Did you know that diets higher in potassium can help control blood pressure by reducing the blood pressure- raising effects of sodium? So, look at our list of foods high in potassium above to help lower blood pressure.

Eye care and complications

Our eyes are important to us at any age. I would ask my patients if they have glasses, do they wear them and when was the last time they had an eye exam. By having good vision, falls can be prevented and it improves the ability to observe surroundings better. By having good vision, you can actually prevent changes in mental status.

Glaucoma and macular degeneration require care by an optometrist or ophthalmologist, so that appropriate treatment, such as eye drops are prescribed. In addition, when out in the sun, wearing sunglasses with 100% UV protection, and are polarized, will reduce light from entering the eye and affecting the retina over time. Especially people with blue or light-colored eyes are at an increased risk for macular degeneration because of this.

My mother-in-law had a "freckle" on her right retina, thought to be melanoma. She lived in the Florida Keys and was exposed to bright light and reflective waters for many years. Back then, there was little knowledge of sun exposure to the eyes. She has bright blue eyes and did not wear sunglasses all of those years.

If the person you care for is having trouble with their vision, consider that they may have cataracts. As you know, cataracts will need surgical treatment to replace the lens in the eye. Sooner or later, we will all develop cataracts if we live long enough. Some trauma to the eye can lead to early cataract surgery, such as a retinal detachment surgery a few years earlier.

It is also important to get a dilated eye exam at least yearly, especially if you have a history of hypertension and diabetes. When the pupil of the eye is dilated, the eye doctor can see to the back of the eye to examine the retina and the macula. There he/she can find if there have been any longstanding medical problems. Blindness can occur for a number of reasons, so get an eye exam yearly.

Conjunctivitis (Pink Eye)

Conjunctivitis is an irritation (inflammation) of the clear membrane that covers the white part of the eye (the conjunctiva) which can become red or pink in color. The person complains that the eye is itchy, tearing, is sensitive to light and he may see some clear drainage near the corner of the eye. Sometimes having a cold can also lead to the virus being spread to the eyes. Conjunctivitis is very contagious due to contact, so good hand washing is key.

There is a proper way to instill eye drops. The most important thing to remember is NEVER to touch the eye with the tip of the eye drop bottle! If this happens, the bottle becomes contaminated, and the infection can now spread to the other eye.

First, wash your hands and obtain tissue and the eye drops bottle.

- Have the person tilt her head back slightly
- Hold the lower lid of the affected eye downward.
- Hold the bottle so that one drop falls into the pocket of the lower lid. Tell the person to blink gently, so the drop gets dispersed across the eyeball. Use the tissue to dab any leaking of fluid on the cheek.

Viral conjunctivitis does not get resolved by antibiotics. Sometimes a sample of discharge can be collected and brought to the lab to determine if it is viral or bacterial. If getting a sample is not possible, then treating the condition first as if it were viral is the right thing to do. What we want to do is prevent the viral condition from becoming a bacterial one.

What is the treatment plan?

- Wash hands with soap and water, dry with a paper towel so you can throw it away
- Use a cool, clean washcloth on the eye or eyes 10 to 20 minutes 4 x/day
- Do not share any towels or washcloths as they can spread the infection
- Wipe away any drainage from the eye, better with a disposable cotton ball
- Change and wash the pillowcase every day
- If the person uses mascara or eyeliner, discontinue its use, and consider discarding it getting a new one when the infection is over
- Do not touch the ointment tube or tip of the eye drop bottle to the affected eye. This way, you will stop the spread of infection to the other eye.
- Clean the eyeglasses regularly

Call your HCP if:

- Pain in the eye increases
- The condition does not change after 3 days of doing the above treatment
- The eye redness is spreading
- Vision becomes blurry
- Oral temperature is above 102 degrees F
- Facial pain or swelling around the eye develops
- Eye condition does not improve with any prescribed treatment started

Allergic Conjunctivitis

Allergic conjunctivitis is the most common cause of eye redness which causes itching, swollen eyelids, and watery, bloodshot eyes. This condition is not contagious. Treatment includes over the counter antihistamines such as Zyrtec or Claritin. I do not recommend Benadryl for the older adult due to its effect on the person's mental status, and possible difficulty urinating.

Blepharitis- what is it?

Blepharitis is an eyelid infection, caused by a viral infection that is limited to the upper or lower eyelid. Sometimes you will notice a small pimple near the lower row of lashes, which is where the problem starts. Like any infection that involves the skin, using warm soaks is the first line of treatment.

Night time soaking:

- Use a clean, soft cloth soaked in hot running water, then wring it out well. Apply it directly to the closed eyelid until cool (which happens quickly).
- Rewarm it and continue the application on and off for 5 to 10 minutes.
- Morning eyelash shampoo:
- Use baby shampoo (especially good to do in the shower) and gently apply the shampoo using your fingers and rub the eyelashes gently.
- Then rinse the shampoo off using warm water.

Eyelid Cleansers

There are some eyelid cleansers that you can purchase over-the-counter that have ingredients in them to wash away any irritants near the eye without irritation. Ocusoft plus or Thera Tears are two such products.

Omega 3 (Flaxseed Oil and Fish Oil Tablets):

One gram (1,000 milligrams) taken orally taken twice a day, can help control blepharitis. Thera Tears Nutrition is an Omega 3 supplement formulated for blepharitis.

Blepharitis has been treated with erythromycin ointment, steroid drops, and antibiotics when and if the condition gets severe; but remember, this condition is chronic and cannot be cured. Continue with the lid hygiene and Omega 3 even after your symptoms are resolved.

Dry Eyes

Over 50% of adults in the United States suffer from dry eye syndrome.

Symptoms are:

- Dryness of the eyes
- Blurry vision
- Light sensitivity
- Excessive tearing
- Stinging and burning

How does dry eyes happen?

- This condition is due to an imbalance of salt due to tearing which leaves the salt behind and makes the tears very concentrated.
- Age- Dry eyes are caused by the natural aging process
- Gender- women tend to be more predisposed to this condition due to hormone changes and menopause
- Environmental conditions: smoke exposure, wind, dry climates
- Medical conditions: Rheumatoid arthritis, diabetes, Sjogren's Syndrome (a type of collagen disorder), thyroid disorders and vitamin A deficiency.

How do you treat dry eyes?

- Artificial Tears is a product that is over-the-counter, or any other product with lubricating drops.
- Purchase drops that are one-time use ampules so are discarded after one day
- Reduce the use of the computer as much as possible because you do not blink as much when staring at a computer screen, therefore causing dry eyes.

- Washing your face before bedtime, and gently washing your eyelids to remove bacteria that cause blepharitis and meibomian gland problems (Small glands on the upper eyelid that helps moisturize the eyeball.)
- Use a warm, moist washcloth to closed eyelids for a minute or two.
- Bean bag eye patches warmed in the microwave for 30 seconds and placed on the eyes at night can help the meibomian glands to work better.

Subconjunctival hemorrhage

This is an eye condition that can occur from rubbing the eye, taking blood thinners or having HTN. It appears as a bright red patch appearing in the white of the eye beneath the clear lining of the eye (conjunctivae). The breakage in a blood vessel can also occur after a sudden sneeze, vomiting, straining or recent eye surgery. It will disappear spontaneously in about 2 weeks.

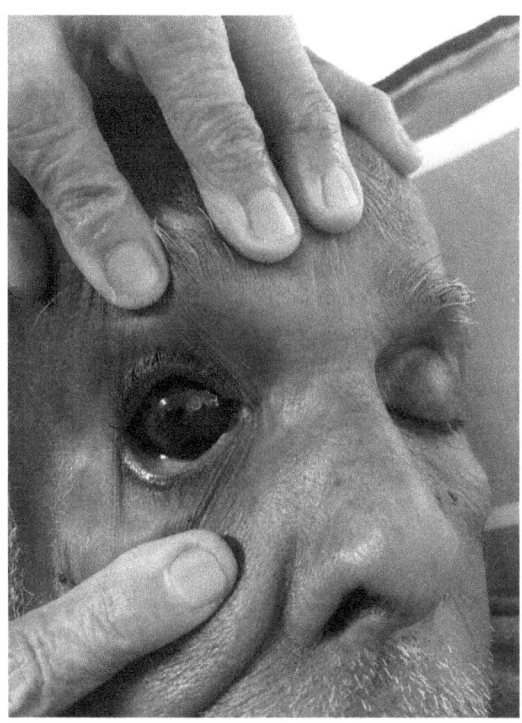

Foot Care Guidelines for Everyone especially over 60

People who lack sensation in their feet or have diabetes can develop foot problems fast. If the foot structure changes such as hammer toes or other bony deformities, these areas can rub on the inside of shoes causing pressure areas.

The serious consequence of foot ulcers can occur if the sensation to feel pain or pressure, usually from poor circulation or nerve damage, is diminished. Therefore, it is important to wear properly fitting shoes. I have changed the type of shoes I wear, lowering the heel height, widening the type of heel for better balance, wearing a wider shoe to reduce ingrown toenails, and ones with good skid surfaces to prevent falling.

Never go barefoot either indoors or outdoors if you are diabetic!

Inspect feet daily- especially if the person is bedridden, does not move in bed, or is paralyzed on one side. That side is the one that has little to no sensation or mobility and is at high risk for skin breakdown. Inspect the soles and between the toes.

Wash your feet daily, testing the water with your elbow to make sure it is not too hot. If the person is in a wheelchair, she can place her feet in a large bowl full of warm water. Do not use a bar of soap but instead, use liquid soap that is gentle, such as Dove soap in a pump container.

Dry areas of the skin should be lubricated with petroleum jelly, Eucerin cream or some other moisturizing cream, but avoid creaming between the toes.

Do not use garters or elastic to hold up stockings, so the skin is not restricted, and circulation is reduced.

Avoid extremes for your feet:

- Do not walk on hot pavement
- Use sunscreen on the top of your feet to prevent sunburn
- Avoid hot water bottles or heating pads to warm cold feet
- Wear socks in bed at night if your feet are cold
- Call a podiatrist to care for your nails, especially if diabetic or have poor circulation. If you cut your own nails, you can cause injury on the skin and have problems with healing.
- If you DO cut your own nails, cut them straight across and avoid rounding the corners
- Do not cut corns or calluses yourself. You can ask your podiatrist how to use a pumice stone

(Diabetes Day-by-Day Foot Care. American Diabetes Association)

- Keep your toes and nails free of dirt or any debris
- Let your HCP know if there is a laceration, blister or sore on your foot immediately
- Placing a pillow to elevate your leg is ok as long as it is from the knee to the heel, not just under the knee
- Do not use tape on your skin, instead use Kling wrap and apply tape over it
- Remember to use an assistive device such as a cane or walker if needed, to prevent injury to your feet when walking
- It is good to walk for exercise and to improve circulation
- Do not smoke. It reduces your circulation and constricts blood flow to the feet

The Diabetic Foot

The best way to take care of and avoid complications of the diabetic foot is to keep blood sugar levels under control. Watch your diet by reducing concentrated sweets, such as candy, cakes, products with sugar; and eat vegetables, fish, drink plenty of water and sugar-free drinks.

Have feet examined as frequently as recommended by your podiatrist.

Sensory neuropathy is the loss of sensation to heat, cold, and pain of the feet. It is imperative that shoes are well-fitting to prevent calluses, corns, and sores that can actually cause ulceration (sores) on the feet.

Autonomic neuropathy- is the loss of nerves that regulate functions that occur without being controlled consciously, like sweating. Cracking, fissures or splits in the skin or foot ulcers can occur when the sweat glands are not working well.

Tinea Pedis- also known as "Athlete's Foot" appears either around the toes and soles of the feet. Symptoms of tinea pedis involve scaling, itching and sometimes, blisters. (see the section under fungal dermatitis below)

Onychomycosis- is a fungal infection under the toenail. The nail can appear patchy yellow or black. It can be painful, and the infection can spread if not treated.

Charcot Joint Disease

This condition results from the destruction of the bones of the feet. Charcot foot happens mostly to diabetics who have a lack of sensation in the feet, causing a change to the foot bones. The foot becomes shortened and deformed, needing a specialized shoe made by an orthotic specialist.

Here are some symptoms:

- Swelling of the foot
- Increased skin temperature of the foot

- Redness in the involved area
- Lack of sweating in the involved area resulting in dry skin
- Structural changes in the foot

What are the risk factors?

The diabetic who cannot feel pain in the foot may develop this condition. He may experience an injury to the foot and not even know it. Instead of resting the foot, the diabetic continues to walk on it. This causes a further injury that may lead to the possible destruction of the bones and joints; hence, greater injury. Twists and sprains may also occur.

How would you know you have charcot foot?

A physical exam, especially by your podiatrist, review of your symptoms and x-rays would lead to this diagnosis.

How do you treat charcot foot?

Daily foot inspection is key. Other devices to protect the foot is rest, use of the wheelchair, a cast, or crutches. You may require surgery, especially if the foot arch collapses. The fusion of the bones may be required. This condition changes everything, so make sure to see your podiatrist regularly for a full foot inspection.

Neuropathic/Diabetic Ulcer

Again, due to lack of sensation in the foot, you may not know you stepped on a nail or hurt the foot. Due to the reduction of blood flow to the diabetic foot, a wound or cut on the foot can get worse very quickly. The cut can turn into an ulcer. Neuropathy is damage to the nerves that give us a sensation. You can lose sensation to heat, cold, or pain. The blood circulation is usually impaired thereby slowing down healing.

What are some of the causes of a neuropathic/diabetic ulcer?

- High blood sugar
- Nerve damage
- Smoking
- Dry and cracked skin
- Being overweight
- Poor circulation
- Athlete's Foot
- Shoes that do not fit

What are some helpful hints to prevent neuropathic/diabetic ulcers?

- Work on controlling your blood sugar
- Wear socks with no seams
- Always wear socks with shoes
- Have your feet checked at each HCP visit
- Never go barefoot
- Gently apply lotion wherever you feel dry or flakiness on the feet
- Wash and check your feet EVERYDAY
- Cut your toenails only if your HCP says it is ok

What can you do if you notice a foot ulcer?

- Make sure to get early treatment to assure quick healing of the wound
- Control infection and pressure relief is important
- Work on eating a healthy diet
- Be active at least 30 minutes a day
- Keep an eye on your blood sugars daily
- Do not skip your diabetes medications

How to change your bandage:

- Wash your hands with soap and water for at least 20 seconds
- Collect your supplies- Kling wrap, tape, gloves, measuring tape, dressing for the wound on a table
- Get into a comfortable position
- Place a large plastic bag or cover on your bed or chair to protect it
- Apply gloves
- Gently unravel the gauze to loosen the dressing
- Gently remove the entire dressing and place it into the plastic bag
- Remove the soiled gloves and discard them into the bag
- Inspect the ulcer and measure it. Look for odor, color, drainage, and amount. Look at the wound bed for any changes
- Reapply a new pair of gloves
- Open all bandage packages
- If there is a cream to apply to the wound, apply it to the dressing, not directly to the wound
- Clean the wound gently as per your HCP
- Reapply the clean dressing
- Make sure the Kling wrap is applied loosely
- Apply tape to the Kling wrap, not the skin
- Report to HCP if wound looks bigger, is swollen, or has more drainage

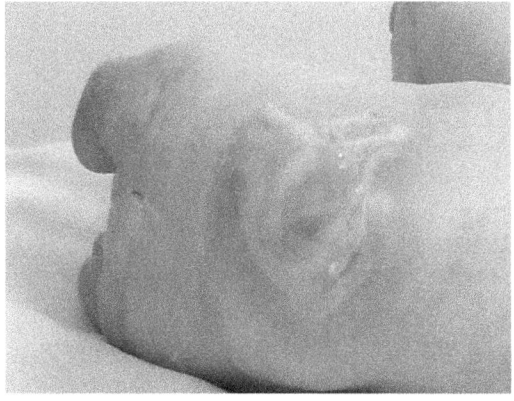

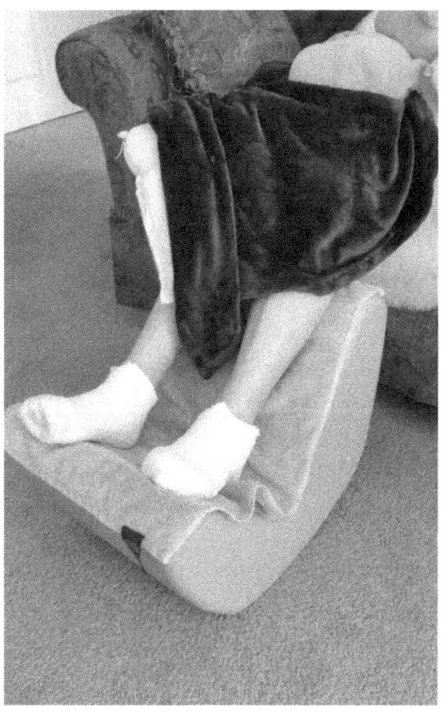

Support for feet

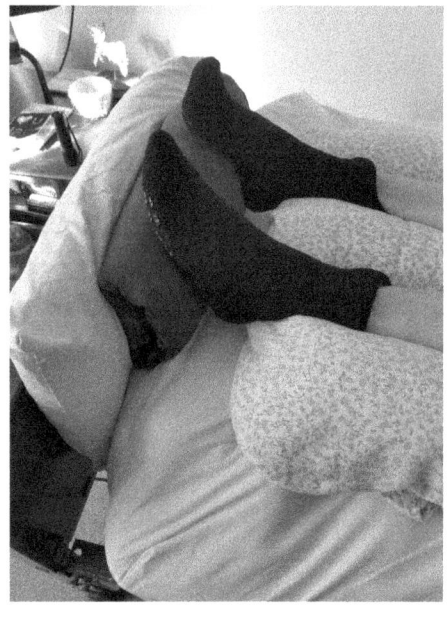

Foot board to help prevent foot drop

Fractures

There are all types of fractures- non-displaced, displaced, comminuted, etc. It is important to rule out a fracture after a fall to determine how bad the fracture is, or if there is one at all. There are companies that do come to the home and can do an x-ray. You would need a prescription from your HCP.

Some fractures require surgery with plates, screws or replacement parts. Some require a sling or just time to heal- usually 4- 6 weeks. Unfortunately, there is usually pain involved, and with that, there is limited mobility of the body part. The person then, requires help, even to comb her hair, or use the walker. PT and OT can be ordered through your HCP to provide professional guidance and therapy during the healing stage.

Taking care of the level of pain is imperative so that the patient can continue with activities of daily living. She may need only Tylenol extra strength 650mg twice a day, or maybe a prescription that is stronger like Tramadol. This medication is an opioid and can become addicting, so use only for a short period of time. It can be ordered 37.5mg with Tylenol in it and used temporarily as the bone heals. Talk with your HCP and be careful when using NSAIDS (Advil, Motrin, Aleve) in the older adult as these medications can cause stomach upset if not taken with food and can be harmful to the kidneys.

If the person that has fallen and has hit her head, she may need a skull and cervical x-ray. If symptoms persist, the x-ray may be repeated in 7 to 10 days to assure a hairline fracture has not been overlooked.

It is important that the person reports to his HCP if he has:

- Pain that is increasing in the neck
- Difficulty swallowing or breathing
- Difficulty walking
- Developed numbness, weakness, or movement problems in the arms or legs
- Developed problems with walking

Fungal Dermatitis (Candidal Intertrigo)

This skin eruption is present mostly in warm, dark, moist areas where there are skin folds: under breasts, armpits, and groin areas. It can also be present in the mouth, mostly on the tongue. The fungus thrives on sweaty areas such as feet where it is called athlete's foot. It appears as a scaly, itchy, burning area on the sole of the foot or between the toes.

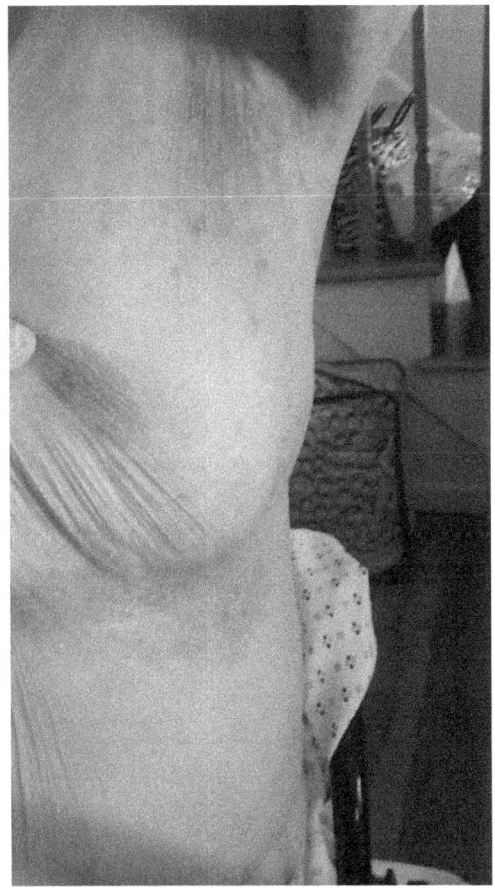

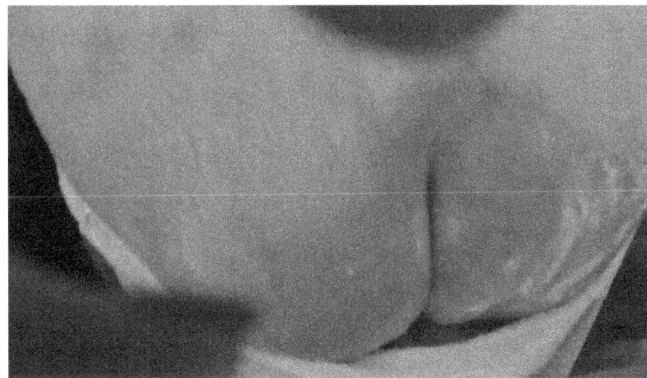

Fungal rash on buttocks

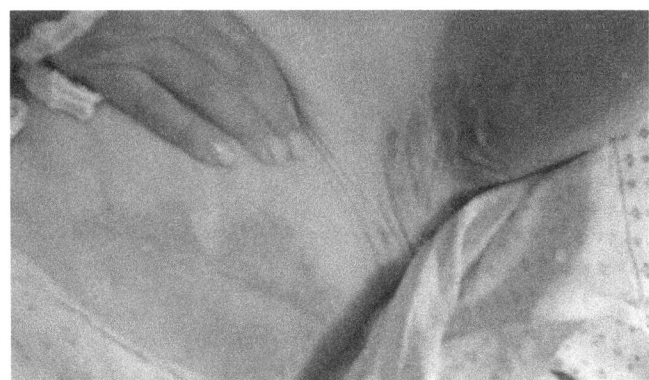

Fungal rash under armpit and in fold

The fungus can be spread from person to person, so it is important to wear gloves and wash your hands after exposure. Another form of fungus is ringworm. These rashes are circular, red, flat, scaly sores.

How to treat fungal rashes:

- First, it is important every day to clean the areas especially skin folds and let the area dry completely
- Light powdering (put a little cornstarch or antifungal powder such as Tinactin), on your gloves
- Gently clap hands together then apply the light powder on your hands to the skin fold
- Avoid using the powder like a "saltshaker" as it cakes the powder if too heavily applied
- There are over-the-counter creams, including Lamisil, Monistat, and Lotrimin that are antifungal

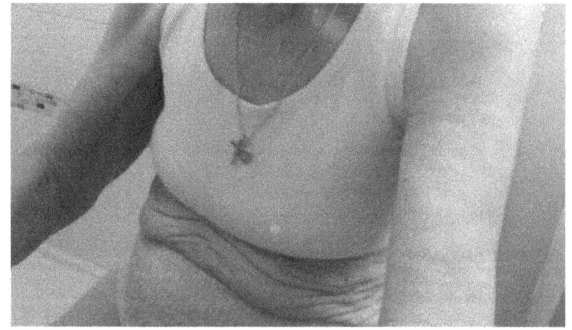

cotton sports bra

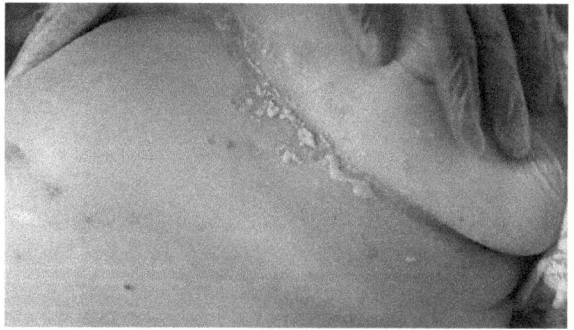

wet cornstarch in breast fold

If the woman does not want to wear a bra, you can cut up small strips of a man's cotton tee shirt into 12 in x 4-inch strips. These strips can be used in all skin folds including abdominal folds. They can be used repeatedly by washing them. Adult diapers can be found online that are washable. Cotton helps the skin breathe and is better for sensitive skin than synthetic materials. Also, wear clothes that are not binding or tight to let the air in. Consider purchasing cotton sports bras to reduce skin-to-skin contact, especially under the breasts.

Yeast Infections (cutaneous candidiasis)

Yeast is another form of fungus. This rash is similar in appearance and symptoms to fungal rashes: red, scaling, itchy; but it is not contagious. Yeast infections are most common in diabetics and obese people. Yeast causes nail infections. Oral thrush is manifested by patches of white on the tongue and inner cheeks. The same treatment is used as above.

Gastrostomy Tube- having one inserted (G-Tube)

This is a major decision that can be an ethical one for the person who is having a gastrostomy tube inserted. For the person who can no longer take in calories orally, without the tube inserted, will eventually lead to death. Death is caused either by constant aspiration of foods into the lungs, or deprivation of calories. It is good for all of us to put our wishes in writing, including if we would want "artificial nutrition." Having a G- tube inserted does not come without its complications: blockage, infection around the stoma (opening), or aspiration. Yes, even when having a G-tube it does not stop the risk of aspiration, which is having liquids go into the lung.

A G-tube is inserted surgically by first making a small incision in the abdomen where the tube is placed. Feedings are given through the tube by two methods: bolus or continuous. The bolus method uses a wide mouth syringe which is connected to the G-tube, allowing a supplement to be poured into the stomach. The higher you hold the G-tube, the faster the supplement pours in so, take your time and go slow. The other method is where the feeding is given through a bag hooked up to a machine, allowing a constant feed of a supplement into the G-tube (like intravenous).

Once a person gets a feeding in a G-tube, he/she needs to sit up no less than 30 minutes with his head high, to prevent the fluid from backing up into the lungs. Sometimes the G-tube can get clogged, and the supplement will not move into the stomach.

To reduce a G-tube clog:

- Disconnect the feeding tube from the pump tubing, or open the clamp on the end of the tube
- Attach a 60 ml (cc) syringe to the feeding tube and pull back on the plunger to remove as much fluid as possible
- Administer 10 ml (cc) of warm water into the tube
- If the blockage does not clear, clamp the tube for at least 5 to 15 minutes, allowing the warm water to soften the clog
- Coke or ginger ale also tends to help dissolve a clog

If the area around the G-tube, called a stoma, gets red or swollen, you can apply Desitin or some other skin barrier cream around the stoma. Calmoseptine also works well for many moist skin areas.

How to apply a dressing around the G-tube:

- Using a 4 x 4 gauze, cut a slit halfway through gauze
- Clean the area around the tube with a wipe or a Periwash spray
- Dry well and apply barrier cream as mentioned above
- Place the cut 4 x 4 around the tube base
- Place paper tape on all sides of the dressing

Hard of Hearing- Is it wax??

Whenever I would visit a patient, I made it a habit to look in their ear canals, and especially when they were having difficulty hearing. It seems that the ears are the most neglected when examining an older person. Without the ability to hear, the person misses the conversation, the news, and happenings around them. This can cause a person with mild dementia to become more disconnected.

If they have a hearing aid, some wax may be lodged in that ear canal, just because the hearing aid holds the wax in the ear. Also, I have found that people who suffer from seasonal allergies tend to make more wax than others.

Another important finding is if a man has hair in the ear or around the outside, the hair tends to catch the wax and makes a "hay and mud" collection causing the wax to stay in the ear. Buying a device that removes hair from the nose with the rotary blade works great for the ear as well.

You know the saying: "don't put anything smaller than your elbow in your ear." That goes for Q-tips. They are supposed to be used on the outside of the ear, and not to be applied INSIDE. By doing so, they become the culprit for wax that can, day after day, slowly build up until you have a blockage in the ear canal.

The person may have to have the wax removed in their HCP's office using an ear lavage device. If there is a little wax, the person can apply a few drops of Debrox in the affected ear every night for a week which may help it gently fall out.

If you wear a hearing aid, leave it out a day after the ear lavage and gently remove any wax from the ear canal with a tissue. This way, the hearing aid does not get oil on it and does not get damaged. If the person is still is not hearing after the wax is removed, check with your local Office of the Aging or google hearing specialists. He may need a hearing aid.

Head Injury

If the person is found on the floor, assume he has hit his head. An unwitnessed fall makes it hard to determine what really happened. Sometimes the person just does not remember, which may mean loss of consciousness, dizziness or fainting that caused the fall. Gently check all extremities for abrasions, and have the person raise arms, and legs. If the person can get up, help him to walk (if they were walking before) to watch for limping, or sounds of groaning as if in pain.

Look for a bump or any sign of bleeding on the scalp. If you see this, do not try to move the person's neck or head, unless they feel they can move it themselves without pain. A concussion is a state of changed mental ability, usually from some trauma to the head. Some symptoms after a head injury are memory difficulties, double vision, headaches, hearing problems, difficulty concentrating, weakness and tiredness. If these symptoms occur, they are common and can last for a few days.

It is important that someone is watching after you for at least the next 24 hours to assure you have no changes in your mental condition. Every 30 minutes for the next three hours after hitting your head, your caregiver should wake you up to check that you have no changes. A cerebral bleed is a real possibility.

What should you do?

- Wrap an ice bag or bag of frozen peas with a wet towel and apply to the scalp for 10 to 20 minutes at a time
- Offer Tylenol or Aleve (if the patient has tolerated this before).
- Have the person rest frequently over the next few days

- If there is a sore or cut on the scalp, apply a thin layer of antibiotic ointment such as bacitracin then a nonstick dressing

Call your HCP if:

- there is increasing pain, swelling or redness around the cut
- report any red streaks leading from the cut
- there is pus (dark yellow drainage) draining from the cut
- you feel any swollen lymph nodes in the neck, armpits or groin
- the temperature is over 100.4 oral

When should you seek immediate medical attention?

- If there is confusion or drowsiness
- If the person cannot be awakened
- If the person has nausea or vomiting
- Dizziness or unsteadiness is getting worse
- There is a clear or bloody discharge from the nose
- Persistent headaches
- Pupils change size and become large covering the colored part (iris) of the eyes
- Severe, persistent headaches not improved with Tylenol

What is post concussive syndrome?

If the person has suffered from a concussion, she may complain of a mild headache or just not feeling well.

She may have:

- changes in the ability to solve problems or concentrate
- a headache
- a change in personality

- a loss of taste or smell
- a change in your ability to walk

Call 911 if:

- You notice twitching, jerking or is having a seizure
- You suddenly cannot stand up or walk
- You lost consciousness
- You are confused, cannot remember where you are
- If you start to vomit and do not stop after 2 hours
- You have headaches that are getting worse
- Your vision is changing
- You notice cool liquid coming out of the nose

Hypercholesterolemia- Do you need to be on a statin at 90?

Hypercholesterolemia or high cholesterol becomes more common as we age. It can be inherited, but also is due to an unhealthy lifestyle. Lack of exercise over the years and eating foods high in fat and salt can be contributors to this condition. There are no symptoms, but by getting a fasting lipid test will determine your numbers for total cholesterol, high-density lipoprotein (HDL) and low-density lipoprotein (LDL), as well as triglycerides.

The one concerning question I had was by the time they had reached 80 or so, is there any true benefit to staying on a statin? I always look at their medical history to decide this. If they have had open heart surgery, diabetes, or history of a stroke, they are advised to stay on the statin.

Risk factors that can increase bad cholesterol:

Poor Diet:
- Eating a high saturated diet consisting of animal products, trans fats found in baked cookies and crackers, and red meat, full- dairy foods like half and half cream in your coffee.

Obesity:
- Having a body mass index (BMI) of 30 or greater

Lack of exercise:
- By exercising, your HDL, which is the good cholesterol, increases while making the LDL become larger "size A" instead of "B" for "bullet," making it less harmful

Smoking:
- By smoking cigarettes, the linings of the blood vessels become more susceptible to accumulating fatty deposits. Smoking can also lower your HDL or good cholesterol

Age:
- The liver changes as we age, becoming less able to remove LDL cholesterol

Diabetes:
- This disease makes us more at risk for elevated cholesterol and heart disease. It increases the very low-density lipoproteins (VLDL) and HDL. Artery linings also get damaged.

What are the complications of having high cholesterol?

Chest Pain:
- If your arteries are getting plaque from cholesterol, so is your heart's arteries. Angina is chest pain as a symptoms of coronary artery disease.

Heart Attack (Myocardial Infarction):
- If a plaque breaks away, it can take off, and then block off an artery in the heart. When the blood flow stops in this artery, you can have major damage to parts of the heart muscle which is called "heart attack."

Stroke:
- The plaque does not travel to the heart but to the brain where it causes damage there

Prevention

- Eat a low- salt diet concentrating on the good foods: fruits, vegetables, and whole grains
- Limit the number of animal fats
- Lose extra pounds and maintain a healthy weight
- Exercise most of the days for 30 minutes
- Manage stress
- Quit smoking
- Drink alcohol in moderation

Coronary Artery Calcium Scan

This test is a special type of CT scan that looks for calcified plaque in the coronary arteries. According to Health.harvard.edu, "findings from large studies link higher calcium scores to a higher risk of a heart attack or stroke."

My Total cholesterol was 260 and my LDL was 160. Insurance did not pay for this test, but I wanted to know based on this test, whether I needed to be on a statin. The score ranges from 1 to 1000, and mine came back as "10". This meant I had a very low cardiac heart disease risk. I opted not to take a statin.

(See the video about the coronary calcium risk test on "Caregiver Success")

Hypertension

What is hypertension? We know it is common in some families, and also happens as we get older. We also know from commercials about medications to treat it and how important it is to control it. Hypertension (HTN) is defined as having a blood pressure of 140/90 mmHg (millimeters of Mercury pressure) of over 140 systolic (top number) and/or over 90 diastolic (bottom number). Example: 140/90. The top number reflects the force of the blood in your vessels when your heart pumps, and the bottom number shows the force of blood in your vessels when your heart is between beats.

Hypertension, also called essential hypertension is defined as a long-term condition where there is an elevation in the pressure of the arteries. The more the heart pumps, and the narrower the arteries become, the higher the blood pressure. You can have HTN for years with no symptoms until a clinician finds it by checking your blood pressure. With high blood pressure, the risk for stroke and heart attack increases, depending on how long and how high the numbers have been. Other complications are an aneurysm, heart failure, weakened blood vessels in the eyes and kidneys, and trouble with memory and dementia.

These medical conditions occur for a number of reasons. As the blood presses against an artery with too much force, the arterial wall loses its stretching ability thereby causing the walls to thicken and the passageway for the blood narrows. Over time, damage to arterial walls can occur loosening plaque and forming clots. A clot can block blood flow in an artery.

Arterial walls can weaken from the force of blood on them causing the walls to break with leakage of blood into nearby tissues causing cell death. This is called an aneurysm.

Symptoms of HTN but are usually when the readings are life-threatening:

- Headache
- Shortness of breath
- Nosebleeds

Secondary hypertension is caused by other factors:

- Obstructive sleep apnea
- Kidney problems
- Adrenal gland tumors
- Thyroid problems
- Certain medications: birth control, cold remedies with Sudafed in them

Risk factors for HTN:

- Age:
  Men are commonly diagnosed with HTN before the age of 65; and women after 65
- Race:
  African heritage is more likely than whites to get HTN
- Family History:
  HTN tends to run in families
- Being overweight or obese:
  The more you weigh, the more blood you need to supply oxygen and nutrients to the tissues. Since the volume of blood circulating increases in the blood vessels, so does the pressure on the arterial walls.
- Being inactive:
  If you are inactive, your heart rate is higher, which causes your heart to work harder causing a stronger force on your arteries.

- Using tobacco:
  Smoking and chewing tobacco give immediate rise to your blood pressure, but the chemicals in the tobacco can damage the arterial walls.
- Too much salt in your diet:
  Eating foods with too much salt causes fluid retention, hence increasing blood pressure
- Too little potassium in your diet:
  Potassium helps balance the amount of sodium in your cells, which increases blood pressure
- Drinking too much alcohol:
  Over time, heavy drinking can damage your heart. Having more than one drink a day for women and more than 2 drinks a day for men may affect your blood pressure. One drink equals 12 ounces of beer, 5 ounces of wine or 1.5 ounces of 80 - proof liquor.
- Stress:
  High levels of stress can lead to a temporary increase in blood pressure. By eating more, drinking more alcohol or smoking more to try to relax, you can also increase blood pressure.
- Certain chronic conditions can increase your risk of HTN:
  Kidney disease, diabetes, sleep apnea

How to take a blood pressure reading:

- It is important when you have your blood pressure checked that both feet are on the floor, the arm being checked is supported by the person taking the blood pressure or on a table at your heart level.
- Have your bp checked in BOTH arms because the one that is higher is the accurate reading.

- The tools used to check blood pressure also have to be right- if you have a small arm and a large cuff is used, you get a lower reading and visa verse.
- First palpate the brachial artery. It is the artery on the inner aspect of the arm where it bends at the elbow.
- Place the blood pressure cuff on the arm with the arrow on the cuff over the brachial artery
- Make the cuff loose enough to be able to insert 2 of your fingers between the cuff and the arm
- Put the stethoscope over the brachial artery and turn the metal wheel clockwise near the bulb
- Pump up the cuff to 180 mm/Hg where the dial on the cuff reaches "180."
- Gently turn the metal wheel counterclockwise so the air in the cuff and the dial starts to go down slowly by 2-3 mm/Hg until you hear the first heart sound- that is called the "systolic" number
- Continue to watch as the dial goes down and simultaneously listen for the LAST sound. That is the diastolic reading
- Now you have the top number/ bottom number= blood pressure reading

(see YouTube at Caregiver Success on "How to take Vital Signs")

You can always purchase a self-monitoring machine such as an Omron machine. You do not need a stethoscope but will need batteries. If you have a large arm do not purchase a regular sized cuff.

Some things you should not do before having your blood pressure checked:

- Do not have any caffeine such as coffee
- Do not eat foods that are high in salt the night before, such as Chinese food
- Avoid high sodium foods such as shellfish

Checking your blood pressure in a pharmacy on one of their machines may not always be accurate. Be sure to check those readings with the ones you have done at the HCP's office. If you are prescribed a blood pressure-lowering medication, it is important to take it every day and not skip, or run out. Some blood pressure-lowering medications, such as Metoprolol should not be stopped abruptly.

Respirate Blood Pressure Lowering Device:

This is a device you can purchase online for about $85. The device actually teaches you how to slow your breathing, which causes dilation of blood vessels, hence, lowering your blood pressure. You wear headphones which has a voice telling you how to breathe. The first phase (Breathing Exercise Phase) takes about 15 minutes. By listening to different tones, you are directed to either breathe in or breathe out. You need to be patient and keep a log of the readings. The goal is to remain in a Therapeutic Breathing Zone for 10 minutes. Your breaths will be under 10 breaths per minute. Getting up to a 40-minute session / week for 4-6 weeks' time will help you lower your blood pressure naturally.

My son, Travis, was told his blood pressure was too high with readings of 150/95 consistently. I sent him the Respirate device to try, and after two weeks of using it, he was able to get his blood pressure to stay down in the 120/ 62 range. He says it helped him to meditate and calm down as well.

If you can reverse some of your lifestyle habits above, such as stop smoking and lose weight, you can actually be taken off high blood pressure pills!

(See "Low Sodium Foods" under "Eating Healthy for Older Adults")

Lung Disorders

Asthma

This condition is a chronic, (or long-term) disease that inflames and narrows the airways of your lungs. Asthma is considered reversible as opposed to emphysema, which is not. It is not curable but controllable. An asthma attack is when the linings of the airways get swollen causing a wheezing sound preventing air to be inhaled. By taking medications daily and, a bronchodilator as needed, asthma can be well-controlled.

Not all asthma is the same- it is measured on the following questions:

- How many times at night you are awakened because you cannot breathe
- Are you having wheezing, coughing, chest tightness and/or shortness of breath
- How often are you using the rescue inhaler, such as albuterol
- Is asthma preventing normal activities?
- How would you do on a breathing test?

Allergy testing to determine what "triggers" the asthma is good to do.

When using an inhaler with steroids, such as Advair, it is important to rinse your mouth out after use to prevent thrush on the tongue.

Airway remodeling, according to the American Thoracic Society, are changes that occur in both the large and small airways, which includes asthma. What this means is there are changes in airway walls where they get thickened, increased mucus secretions, causing excessive coughing. When I explain to patients what remodeling is, I use the analogy of "rubber bands" tightening around the lungs making it difficult to breathe.

Pulmonary Hypertension (PH)

The U.S. National Library of Medicine defines PH as "abnormally high blood pressure in the arteries of the lungs." In simpler terms, the heart has to pump blood with oxygen through the lungs but has to work harder due to narrowed blood vessels. Sometimes the blood oxygen levels are low, so supplemental oxygen is needed.

Bronchiectasis

This lung disease is caused by smoking, of which the lungs are inflamed. The person has a chronic cough with a large amount of phlegm which gets trapped in the lungs, causing shortness of breath and fatigue. Oxygen therapy is a common treatment for this disorder.

Lung Cancer

Cancer in the lung causes changes to some of the tissues which cause abnormal functioning. Delivery of oxygen to the tissues is more difficult. According to WebMD, oxygen therapy is used to improve comfort for the patient with lung cancer but does not treat the disease.

Black Lung

This disease is caused by excessive inhalation of coal dust from mines. Low-dose oxygen therapy can help reduce the symptoms of fatigue, and breathlessness.

Chronic Obstructive Pulmonary Disease (COPD)

This disease is called obstructive because it restricts air flow and causes long-term breathing problems. COPD is considered to worsen over time. Common symptoms are shortness of breath, and coughing with sputum production. The person complains that his chest feels tight, may have a wheezing sound when he breathes. As the condition worsens, the person takes on a "tripod" stance, leaning on a table with hands down, just to catch a breath.

Here are some symptoms of COPD:

- Cough that does not go away
- Coughing up a lot of mucus
- Shortness of breath, especially with exercise
- Wheezing
- Chest tightness

You can have COPD even if you don't have symptoms. Only your HCP can assess you for lung disease by performing a breathing test called spirometry. Exposure to air pollution and family history of the disease are some of the causes. There is no cure for COPD, but treatment and lifestyle changes can help control your symptoms. Some may not want to see an HCP because they may think the symptoms are due to age, smoking, lack of exercise or a virus.

Many people may delay seeking care because they may be ashamed that they caused the condition because they smoked. Or that they are afraid about getting bad news, nothing can help them, or they do not want to be lectured about bad habits.

Managing COPD requires taking your medications including inhalers and nebulizers as directed. The nebulizer cup needs to be cleaned after each use. It is important not to run out of medication or skimp on medication to make it last longer. Using the air conditioner to keep the air pure and less humid helps to breathe easier. It is important to stay inside when there is pollution or poor air quality. It is important to drink plenty of fluids to keep the mucus loose.

Chronic bronchitis and emphysema are under this umbrella term, COPD. Tobacco smoking, air pollution and a small part of genetics play a part in the cause of COPD. Over time with this exposure, the lung tissues become inflamed and the airways narrow, making breathing more difficult. One test done to determine the diagnosis is a lung function test. COPD is not reversible, as asthma is. Treatments include smoking cessation, vaccinations (such as Prevnar 13, 20, influenza), bronchodilators, steroids and, sometimes, low-dose oxygen. A nebulizer is very beneficial for this person, as they inhale medications that improve lung function, therefore, quality of life.

Pulmonary rehabilitation is a program that can help to breathe better. It could help with maintaining fitness and improving breathing. Some exercises recommended are walking, stationary bicycling, water exercise and simple aerobics.

It can be difficult performing some tasks when you have COPD. Do things slowly, put items you use all the time in places of easy reach, wear loose clothing, and shoes that are easy to put on. Use a reacher to pick up items and use a cart on wheels to move things around.

Lymphedema

We have two sets of circulation: blood and lymphatic. The lymphatic system circulates to remove bacteria from the bloodstream to help maintain a healthy body. It is part of our cardiovascular system. When the volume of lymphatic fluid increases, the fluid accumulates. Lymphedema can occur in only one leg. The skin can get thick, and the leg can change shape. Lymphedema can also occur on the arm, especially after a mastectomy where lymph nodes are removed from the armpit. This condition reduces quality of life due to the heaviness of the limb and difficulty for performing regular ADL's.

There is no cure, unfortunately, but physical therapy could assist with massage of the legs to move the lymphatic drainage upward, application of elastic wraps and teaching how to use compression boots or compression sleeves. The Flexi touch system is an advanced intermittent pneumatic compression device (lymphedema pump) used by many patients to self-manage lymphedema and non-healing venous ulcers. This device is worn at night and is portable resulting in better compliance. To find out more about the Flexi touch system, call Tactile Medical at 833-382-2845 or go to www.tactilemedical.com to learn more.

Medication Tips

Many older adults have more than one provider. They are to provide a list of medications they are taking whenever they go to see an HCP. The list should include OTC remedies as well as prescription medications. Keeping this list in your wallet, will help you remember everything you are taking when you need to present it. They are also providing their pharmacy for a new prescription.

Now that I am a Medicare recipient, I am navigating this system just like you. In the last year, I have been prescribed two expensive medications. I tried the drug programs such as Good RX and Single Care, as well as the mail away program from my advantage plan for a better price. They all could not beat the plan I found through the state of CT called ArrayRx.

I was at the doctor's office, for instance, and was ordered a cream that I would need to use twice a week indefinitely. The doctor asked me who my pharmacy was to call it in. I said I will find out the best deal and she could send the prescription there. I made the above calls from the waiting room and found out that if I go through Array RX using my zip code and the drug name, dosage and frequency, I could find a pharmacy near me for the cheapest price. The prescription would have been $400.00 but it was $9.95 for a month supply. I am learning how to be a better advocate for myself, even as a provider. Be sure to check by googling prescription discount plans in your state to find out if there is a discount drug plan there.

(see my YouTube video on Caregiver Success "How to get the best buy for your prescription.")

Polypharmacy is when excessive or inappropriate medications are ordered. Being on multiple medications over time and with age, causes adverse drug side effects. A third of hospital admissions are due to adverse drug effects and are preventable.

Medications Older Adults Should Avoid

1- Non-Steroidal Anti-inflammatory Drugs (NSAID)

These medications are used for inflammation and arthritis. For the older adult, they should be used only short-term with a maximum of two weeks, and always take with food.

They can cause liver and kidney problems, abnormal bleeding, stomach ulcers, allergic rashes, high blood pressure and lead to unnecessary hospitalization.

Examples: Aleve, Motrin, Ibuprofen, Advil

2- Digoxin in a dose higher than 0.125mg due to increased risk of toxicity

3- Some diabetic drugs: glyburide (Diabeta, Micronase), Diabenese. These medications have long half-lives which means it takes a long time for the drug to leave the bloodstream leaving low blood sugars longer.

4- Muscle relaxants: Flexeril (cyclobenzaprine), Robaxin (methocarbamol), Soma (carisoprodol) These medications cause dry mouth, dizziness, muscle weakness, loss of appetite.

5- Certain medications for anxiety and/or insomnia: (Valium, Xanax, Sonata, Ambien) These medications are highly addicting

6- Anticholinergic drugs are drugs that work on neurotransmitters in the brain and include anti-histamines for allergies, skeletal muscle relaxants, antipsychotics, urinary incontinence, and overactive bladder. (Detrol, Benadryl, Amitriptyline, Ditropan, Zyprexa) Side effects include drowsiness, confusion, drug mouth, constipation

7- Pain relievers like Demerol, Percocet, and Oxycodone. These drugs are highly addicting and of the class "opioids."

8- Avoid estrogen pills: causes blood clots
(Adapted from The American Geriatrics Society April 2012)

Disposal of unneeded or outdated medications:

We know there is an epidemic of drug abuse. Partly when medications such as Oxycodone which was given to you after your hip replacement two years ago, is still in the medicine cabinet, there is the chance that someone in your family who is drug seeking will find it.

Once a year (or more often if necessary), gather all medications that you no longer take. Empty them from their bottles and put them in a sealable plastic bag. Mix them with either coffee grounds or something else that is unappealing, such as kitty litter. They can then be disposed of in the garbage. There is also a product called Deterra drug deactivation system. It is a package that can be purchased on line. You pour your medications into the packet, fill the pouch halfway with warm water, wait 30 seconds, seal the pouch tightly, gently shake and dispose of in normal trash.

Some of your local Police stations are taking unwanted medications as well. Just remove the label off the bottle and hand them in. You will be glad you did. Proper disposal of unused drugs saves lives and protects the environment. For more information on prescription drug abuse, go to www.dea.gov or www.justthinktwice.com

For disposal of sharps, you can go on www.stericycle.com, click on your state, put in your zip code to find out how to safely dispose of sharps.

I want to show you how to crush a pill: take two small spoons
Place the pill in one of the spoons
Place the other spoon on top of the pill
Push the two spoons together

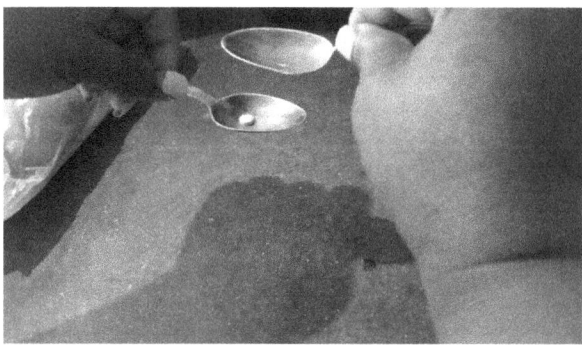
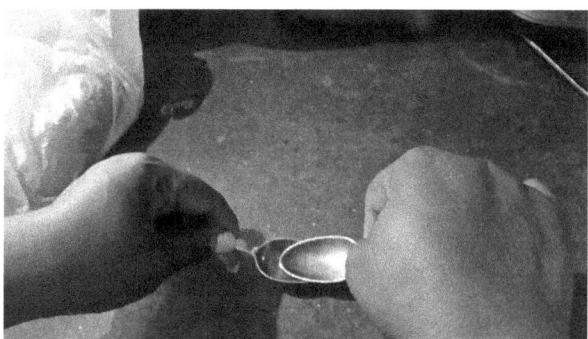

If the person you are caring for is taking Sinemet for Parkinson's disease, I tell her to have the first pill of the day near her bedside to take before arising in the morning. The rationale is that people complain of less morning stiffness when the medication is taken before they start to walk around. It also prevents falling or choking on morning medications or food due to general neurological stiffness.

Lotrisone- this is a combination of cortisone 1% and a nystatin cream. This is a prescription cream that is not cheap. It is used for areas that are reddened, usually on the buttocks or in the folds. The cortisone base helps with the redness, and the nystatin reduces the fungal part of the rash. By combining the cortisone cream and nystatin 1:1, which are both over the counter, you have made your own Lotrisone cream.

Medications are taken more consistently if you have a pill box and fill it up once a week. Depending on how many times a day you take medication, you can get up to a 4 time-a-day box. There are some devices that can remind you it is time to take your medicine for those who are more forgetful. I found this electronic pill box online called MedFolio. It has the ability to tell you that it is time to take your medication.

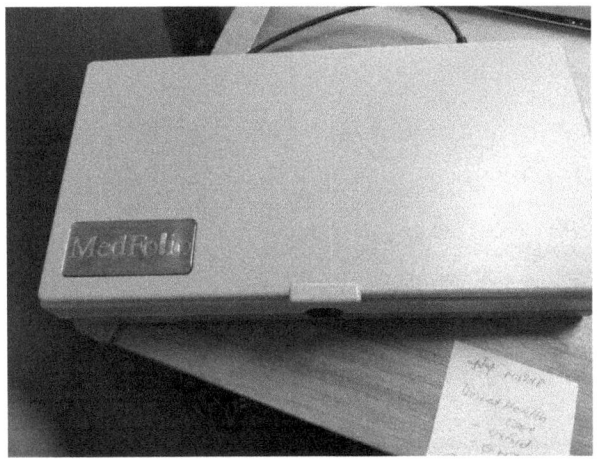 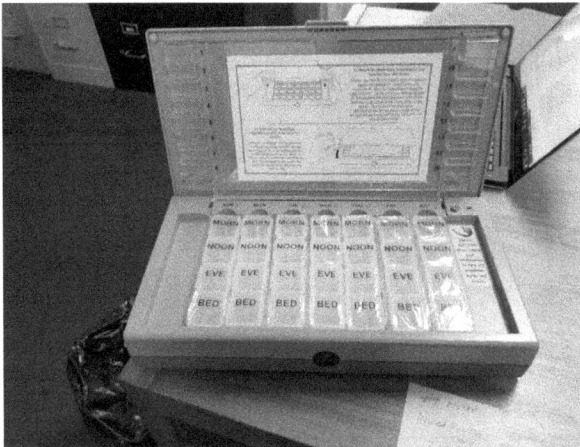

For those that have trouble with medication compliance, Pill Pak could be the solution. A pharmacy works directly with your HCP to order your medications, including insulin, inhalers and prescriptive creams. Medications are pre-packaged based on the frequency they need to be taken and labeled so that you know what medications are in the package. The service is free, and the packages of medications are delivered right to your doorstep. Check out www.pillpak.com to learn more.

Mental Health Conditions

Mental illness is a real medical problem for many homebound people. Some do not leave home due to fear of people, anxiety of leaving home, due to agitation or dementia. By bringing the program to the home, we are able to get the person out into society to get further help and to assimilate with those around them.

Alcoholism/Addictive Behaviors

Everyone likes to have a good drink now and again, but it does not come without risk if you are taking an antidepressant. With the first drink, you may feel happier and have a better mood, but its overall effect increases symptoms of anxiety and depression. As we get older, we may also be taking medications to help with sleep or pain. These medications can cause a dangerous reaction when taken with alcohol. Some antidepressants cause sedation and drowsiness, and so does alcohol. So, when taken together the effect is intensified.

Alcohol Use Disorders Identification Test (AUDIT) is a questionnaire to screen for excessive drinking and alcohol use disorders. A score of 8 or more is associated with harmful or hazardous drinking. A score of 13 or more in women and 15 or more in men is likely to indicate alcohol dependence.

It is important not to stop the antidepressant so you can have a drink since these medications need to be safely tapered down in order to be stopped. Also, stopping and starting the antidepressant can make the depression worse. If you are feeling more depressed, speak with your HCP about it, because people with depression are at increased risk of substance abuse and addiction. Also, people with depression who need help with trouble sleeping may use alcohol to help them. It may help you fall asleep, but you may wake up in the middle of the night. Be careful with some cough suppressants as they have alcohol in them also, and may not mix with your other medications. (Mayo Clinic June 9. 2017)

Anxiety Disorder

It is normal to feel anxious about new situations or new illnesses, but when you are anxious all of the time, and this feeling keeps you from doing things, it is time to seek help. Social phobia is when the person is overwhelmed in social situations. They are afraid they will not remember names or are ashamed of their appearance.

Generalized Anxiety Disorder (GAD) is when the person is constantly worrying with no cause for it. Older adults with GAD have difficulty concentrating, sleeping or relaxing; and are easily startled. Their symptoms include chest pain, headaches, muscle tension, sweating, frequent trips to the bathroom and feeling out of breath.

Post-traumatic stress disorder can occur after a traumatic event- rape, a car accident, war, natural disasters, such as fire or flood. Sometimes the event is re-lived by the older adult 30 years later when they find themselves helpless again from a new illness. They may display irritability, aggressiveness or nightmares.

Panic disorder is when those with this disorder suffer from sudden attacks of terror, even when sleeping. It is manifested by an episode of up to 10 minutes duration of heart pounding, sweating, dizziness or nausea.

Why should an older adult be concerned about anxiety? Anxiety and depression go hand in hand. They both can be debilitating reducing quality of life and overall health. Also, anxiety is linked to memory loss.

Depression

Depression is the most common mental disorder seniors will face, but is not considered a normal part of aging. Social isolation can cause depression. Depression is also a symptom of dementia that tends to get overlooked. It affects how you feel, think, and handle daily activities, such as sleeping, working and eating. It is thought that most older adults feel satisfied with their lives, even though they have more illnesses or physical problems.

Major depression is an episode that can occur once in someone's lifetime and affect all aspects of daily living. Whereas, a persistent depressive disorder is a depressed mood that lasts for at least 2 years with episodes of major depression with periods of severe or lesser symptoms. Other causes of depression can be genetics, (since it does run in families), a stressful life, personal history of depression when younger, or different brain chemistry.

Another form of depression can be vascular. The person suffers from a lack of blood to the brain due to a restricted blood flow, which can also affect other organs as well. They may be at risk for, or may have, heart disease, or had a stroke. This condition is especially true if there is no family history of depression.

When I performed an Annual Wellness Exam for the over 65 individual, part of the questions asked were about depression. A PHQ-9 depression screen is reviewed with the person asking 10 questions about how they have felt over the last 2 weeks. It also asks if you ever considered committing suicide; and if so, did you have a plan. If the answer is yes, they need to be referred immediately to a Mental Crisis intervention Team.

Dysthymia is a chronic form of depression. The person loses interest in normal day-to-day activities. You may feel hopeless, have low self-esteem and have an overall feeling of inadequacy. You may feel gloomy and not enjoy fun activities. This condition is not as severe as major depression. Using talk therapy and medication can be effective in treating this condition.

Treatments for Depression

Your HCP can assess, after checking some blood work (thyroid, electrolytes, CBC, and urinalysis), if the person needs an antidepressant called an SSRI (Selective Serotonin Reuptake Inhibitor). I would ask the person if there is anyone with depression in the family and if so, what they are taking for medication and is it effective. If they have addictive behaviors, such as excessive drinking or smoking, sometimes we start Wellbutrin instead. These medications take up to 4 weeks to take full effect. They are not to be stopped abruptly but need to be tapered down. Talk therapy is an adjunct to the medication and can help the medication work better.

Prevention of Depression

Regular exercise, eating a balanced diet and finding something you like to do, that gives you purpose can help you avoid depression. Try to prepare for life changes such as retirement or moving from a home you lived in for many years. Stay in touch with your family and friends and let them know when you are not feeling happy. For more information about depression, call the American Psychological Association Support Team at 1-800-374-2721, or Depression and National Alliance for bipolar disorder at 1-800-950 NAMI (6264) or info@nami.org.

Late Onset of Bipolar Disease

- This condition is diagnosed in early adulthood. Late onset bipolar presents with more severe symptoms from acting very down (depressive), to an increase in activities (mania).
- Feeling as if moving is an effort
- Lack of interest in enjoyable activities

- Feeling of no worth or value that they can contribute
- Weight fluctuations
- Agitated pacing and inability to sit still with constant fidgeting
- Social withdrawal
- Being over-demanding with displays of angry verbal outbursts

Symptoms of mania

- Decreased need for sleep
- Acting paranoid
- Moving faster than usual, leading to falls and injuries

Treatment for Bipolar Disease: requires a psychiatric consultation for talk therapy and medication management.

Hoarding

I will never forget my patient, Paul. He was a war veteran who lived alone with his dog. He lived in a 4-room home. Paul saved everything- bags, newspapers, boxes with nothing in them. He made a small path for me so I could come in through the kitchen door and put my medical bag on the top of a pile of papers. Every room was filled up to the top of the windows with only paths to get from room to room.

A hoarding disorder is a persistent difficulty of discarding or parting from possessions because of a need to feel they have to be saved. Hoarding becomes a private behavior. Eventually, the rooms become unusable and unsafe, especially for the older person who may have an unstable gait. Food and trash can be part of the clutter, leading to unsanitary conditions.

What causes this disorder? It is not clear but thought to be possibly caused by genetics or stressful life events. This disorder involves people with the personality of indecisiveness. It tends to run in families. Stressful life events such as divorce, fire, and death of a loved one can fuel this disorder. They have an obsessive component where they feel the need to keep items.

This group of people usually experience other mental disorders, such as depression, anxiety, obsessive-compulsive disorder (OCD) and attention-deficit/hyperactivity disorder (ADHD). There is little that is understood about the cause or how to prevent it — getting treatment when it is noticeable may help the problem from getting worse.

Cognitive behavioral therapy can help you learn how to avoid acquiring more items, organize possessions, and how to de-clutter your home. Treatment involves the assistance of the family, friends, and agencies in your county to help remove the clutter.

Consider working with a de-cluttering company like POSSE Partners, LLC. POSSE stands for

Purge
Organize
Sort
Select
Equalize (maintain without re-cluttering)

Jean Herron, professional organizer says "Less clutter, more you" and "all roads lead to paper." She mentions how you can make a memory box of trinkets from the past, but get rid of the rest. Go to NAPO (National Association for Professional Organizers) to find one near you.

(Check out on YouTube, Caregiver Success- the video on Do You Need to Declutter?")

Psychosis

Psychosis is a change in a mental condition where the person is disconnected from reality. One of my patients told me that they were seeing children playing on the ceiling and heard a loud party in the backyard when these instances did not exist. Sometimes the person would report hearing voices or strange sounds. It can be quite frightening to the individual, and sometimes the person becomes angry, nervous or agitated.

If there is a change in a person's mental status, reach out to your HCP to have the person examined. This change could be due to pneumonia or a urinary tract infection. Blood work that may be ordered: CBC with differential to check for elevated white blood cells showing infection, or perhaps, anemia if the hemoglobin is low; complete metabolic panel to check the kidneys for dehydration; the thyroid (TSH) to see if the anxiety is from a change in the thyroid gland, and vitamin B12, folate and vitamin D to check for deficiencies.

In addition, I worked with a behavioral health group that consisted of a nurse practitioner (NP), social worker, and psychiatric NP. We talk about the patient's symptoms, what the family tells us is going on, and medications such as Zyprexa and Risperidone are considered and tried. As a group, we talked weekly to see what the new medication is doing for the person's behavior and would adjust it based on the report. This process kept the patient in their home, having them receive counseling sessions by phone and having daily medical intervention as needed.

Suicide

In 2017, my father-in-law took his life. He was 87 years old, had lost his driver's license due to poor eyesight as he was "unable to distinguish a weed from a flower" and he felt he had no purpose. He was told that he had an early stage of dementia. He did not want to be a burden on his wife or his seven children.

Like a "tree man" he was still able to climb a ladder, tie a knot, and throw a rope over a strong branch. It was amazing that he was able to do this since he could not lift his arms over his head and had a heart condition. His wife, Mary, and her son Jim were at our home when it happened. It was shocking to all of us, but Mary mentioned that Dad was talking for a while about leaving us, but she did not tell anyone.

I found this incident to be eye-opening. I have had many patients plead with me to "give them something" to end their lives. For Dad to do this because of how he felt about living, it gave him the power to have control over his own destiny. The rippling effect of this act has taken away his birthday, his wedding anniversary and all future memories. We all know that we have our mortality to think about. As a Christian, I do not believe in taking my own life, but Dad was not religious. It took a year for our family to have a memorial for Dad, as Mary was going through the stages of grief and was angry that he left her alone.

I will say, Mary recovered well- she was busy with the "lunch bunch"- friends that are widowed and have become her local family in Florida. She has trusted that God will be loving and forgiving for what her husband has done.

Watch for the Signs of Suicide:

- Suicide attempts
- Previous suicide attempts
- Alcohol and drug abuse
- Statements revealing a desire to die
- Sudden changes in behavior
- Prolonged depression
- Making final arrangements
- Giving away prized possessions
- Purchasing a gun or stockpiling pills

QPR- Question- Persuade- Refer

Question the person about suicide. Do they have thoughts? Feelings? Plans? Don't be afraid to ask.

Persuade the person to get help. Listen carefully. Then say, "let me help." Or, "come with me to find help."

Refer for help. If a child or adolescent, contact any adult, any parent. Or call your minister, rabbi, tribal elder, a teacher, coach or counselor.

To Save A Life….
Realize someone might be suicidal
Reach out. Asking the suicide question DOES NOT increase risk
Listen. Talking things out can save a life.
Don't try to do everything yourself. Get others involved.
Don't promise secrecy and don't worry about being disloyal
If persuasion fails, call your mental health center, local hotline or emergency services
If you believe someone is in the process of making a suicide attempt, call 911. The person is so depressed that he stops eating or gets very thin, talks less, sits in the dark alone, and is easily irritated. Older people may have trouble sleeping or feel tired. When they have heart disease, stroke, or cancer, he/she may have depression.

If you suspect a person you love is thinking of suicide, call the toll-free number for the National Suicide Prevention Lifeline 1-800-273-(TALK) 8255, or 1-800-SUICIDE (784-2433).
Vets4Warriors is 1-855-838-8255,
In Crisis? Text 741741 or call 9-8-8 or 2-1-1.
(information from www.qprinstitute.com)

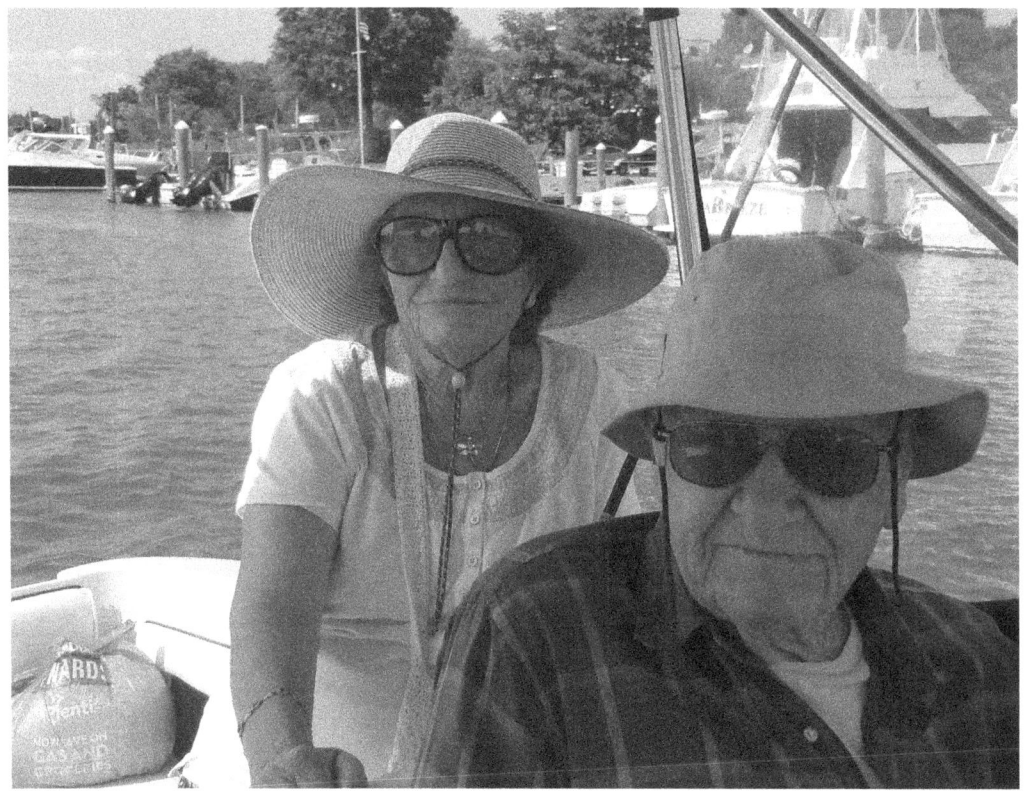

Steve's mother and father, Mary and Don

I worked with a behavioral health integration team consisting of a social worker, psychiatrist and a nurse practitioner, to help our patients with not only their chronic medical conditions but also, their mental health. After developing a behavioral health story of the person, review of blood work, diagnoses, and medications, the psychiatrist will offer medical suggestions. We have a virtual meeting weekly to discuss patient progress. This program has proven to be invaluable for our patients. Check with your HCP if they have such a program that is covered by Medicare.

Matthew 5:4
Blessed are those who mourn, for they shall be comforted.

Obesity in the Older Adult

It is a fact that people with obesity are more likely to develop health problems such as heart disease, diabetes, sleep apnea, osteoarthritis, gall stones, and hypertension. In the U.S. about 40% (9.3 million people) are obese, according to the Centers for Disease Control and Prevention (CDC). In a person over 65, it is difficult to lose weight, as we have limited flexibility and mobility just from common aging problems, such as arthritis.

Obesity is defined as having a BMI (Body Mass Index) over 30. This measurement is calculated by the ratio of height to weight. BMI alone may not be the only screening tool for obesity and considering a person's physical, mental and functional health may be a better approach. Functional health refers to a person's ability to move around and perform ADL's.

Obesity occurs when people eat and drink more calories than they use. Not only is over-eating a factor but lack of sleep, lack of physical activity and side effects from certain medications can cause weight gain. Some illnesses attributed to weight gain are hypothyroidism, Cushing's syndrome, polycystic ovary syndrome and a rare condition called Prader-Willi Syndrome (a rare genetic condition where a person never feels full).

If only we were able to take better care of ourselves over the years so that we could "dance" our way into the "golden years." I have taken care of multiple obese patients who became bedridden due to leg edema, shortness of breath and poor endurance. Over time, it was easier to stay in bed than to get up and move around.

The problem is that it is difficult for the caregiver to clean and position an obese bedridden person, especially if the person cannot assist in her care, such as holding onto the bed railing during cleaning. Her care may require 2 caregivers to achieve results. In addition, skin problems such as fungal rashes occur due to folds in the skin not getting proper cleaned or lack of aeration. Bed sores can occur due to pressure from lack of movement.

Even the loss of a small amount of weight- 5 to 10% of your total body weight – can improve health, according to the CDC. Blood pressure, blood sugar and cholesterol numbers all could be reduced.

What are some tips you can do to lose weight?

- Keep a daily food diary (it helps you see what kind of foods you have been consuming during the day)
- Make small changes to your eating habits: drink more water and slow eating pace down
- Find ways to include healthy habits like taking a walk during the day
- Consider eating a lighter meal at dinner
- Set realistic goals for weight loss

Osteoporosis- what it is and how to prevent it

Osteoporosis is a bone disease that causes bones to become weak and more likely to break due to a decrease in bone density and thickness. It is also known as "thin bones, "low bone density" and "metabolic bone disease."

Our bones are in a constant state of change and replacement through our early youth. Usually, by the time we are in our mid-20's, we have reached our bone peak. As we age, bone mass is lost faster than it was made. What we did in our youth can determine what our bones will look like later in life.

Who is at the greatest risk for osteoporosis?

- White and Asian women after menopause
- Family history- especially if your mother or father experienced a hip fracture
- Men and women who are small framed

Estrogen is a hormone we produce throughout our lives. When a woman reaches menopause, the estrogen is no longer released from the ovaries. This estrogen has been the protection to prevent bone thinning.

A bone density test is done especially after menopause to determine whether there has been bone loss. And if there has, then measures can be taken to help build back bone before osteoporosis occurs.

Obese or overweight women have a lesser chance of developing osteoporosis because the fatty tissue retains estrogen long after menopause occurs. Excess weight has been known to increase the risk of fractures in the arm and wrist. (Mayo Clinic 2018)

There are medical conditions that can increase the risk of osteoporosis:

- poor calcium absorption due to surgery to remove a part of the stomach rheumatoid arthritis
- thyroid problems (where too much thyroid hormone can cause bone loss) overactive parathyroid or adrenal glands
- Lupus
- Cancer
- Multiple myeloma
- Inflammatory bowel disease
- Celiac disease
- kidney or liver disease.

Lifestyle habits like chronic smoking, being underweight, drinking more than 3 alcoholic drinks a day increases osteoporosis risk. A sedentary lifestyle, such as a sit-down job, or being bedridden or no longer walking reduces the weight-bearing action of actually stepping on your feet with all your weight. This action does help keep our bones dense. Some other causes are high protein intake, vitamin D deficiency and prolonged use of steroids.

Carbonated beverages were thought to have a high relationship with bone loss. The fact is that people tend to substitute beverages high in calcium, like milk and fortified juices with carbonated beverages, which may affect the total amount of calcium intake. Some brands of seltzer contain up to 150 mg of calcium; and some mineral waters are rich in calcium (according to Karen Alexander, OWS Ackerman Cancer Center 9/9/16)

There are medications used for seizures, gastric reflux (heartburn), cancer and transplant rejection that have been associated with increased risk of osteoporosis.

Understanding Your Bone Density Test Results

A bone density test is a low- dose x-ray known as a DEXA scan. The test indicates how dense your bones are and whether you are at risk for a fracture. When you have the test done, the lumbar spine and the left hip are x-rayed to check the thickness of your bones. The test is very simple and painless and should be done once to every other year, after menopause.

Your HCP will give you a prescription for the test, and make an appointment with a radiology or a Women's center (where mammograms are also done). Wear sweat pants and loose clothing. The test takes about 10 minutes to complete.

According to the U.S. Preventive Services Task Force, every woman over the age of 65 should have a baseline bone density test done. And women are twice as likely as men to suffer from broken bones because of osteoporosis (National Osteoporosis Foundation).

Some clinical signs of osteoporosis:

- Humpback or stooped posture (kyphosis)
- Bone fractures that sometimes occur spontaneously and without falling
- Back pain caused by a fractured or collapsed vertebra
- Loss of height over time
- Hip pain
- Inability to bear weight in the hip
- Shortened, externally rotated leg

Men can also develop osteoporosis if their testosterone level is low. A simple blood test can help you determine this. If a man is treated for prostate cancer, the medication used to treat it, also reduces testosterone, leading to bone loss. If the testosterone is low, taking the hormone will help build bone. Fosamax, testosterone therapy and parathyroid hormone therapy are treatments to slow bone loss and reduce fractures for men.

What you can do to strengthen your bones:

If your bone density result shows osteoporosis: T score greater than -2.5, then medical treatment should be started. Going to an Osteoporosis Center or seeing an endocrinologist can determine the root cause of the disease. Having a bone density between 0 and -1.5 means osteopenia or thinning of the bone; this means you are not at osteoporosis yet and can reverse your bone density by changing lifestyle habits, taking certain vitamins, and exercising with weight bearing.

Eating a well-balanced Diet

Women under the age of 63 who ate lots of fruits, vegetables, fish and whole grains were less likely to have a hip fracture. It is also important to eat foods rich in calcium, magnesium, and potassium, especially for women over the age of 69. Avoid drinking cola carbonated beverages.

There are two tests that can tell you if you have a balance problem. First, walk with one foot right in front of the other -heel to toe, and walk in a straight line, and the other is to stand on one foot for 30 seconds. If you cannot do either test, it would be good to seek physical therapy to help you improve balance.

Strength training is a way to help make your muscles stronger and maintain strength and flexibility. Visit the Mayo Clinic website: Osteoporosis Insight (12/5/18) for a video about exercises you can do, either as the person in the bed, or the caregiver. Taking classes for Tai Chi- the ancient art of balance and movement can help reduce the risk of falling.

Treatment for osteoporosis

Depending on how thin the bones are, there are multiple treatments to help reverse or slow down osteoporosis. Fosamax is a well - known medication (biphosphonate) and should not be taken more than 5 years, as it is known to have no further effects after that time. (Mayo Clinic 2018).

   Adult women and men over the age of 71 should take 1200 mg calcium per day.

(Go to YouTube, Caregiver Success and watch my video "Osteoporosis- learn about it")

(Check out on the Mayo Clinic Marketplace site "Mayo Clinic Guide to Preventing and Treating Osteoporosis.")

Oxygen Deprivation

My father was sleeping a lot, seemed a little confused and was just "off". When I checked his oxygen level with my oximeter, it was low at 90. Our oxygen level on an oximeter can be up to 100%. This is a device that checks the person's oxygen level by placing the oximeter on a finger. Some fingers can be cooler than others and so, it may be difficult to get an actual reading. By trying different fingers, you may be more successful in getting a reading. It is a starting point for determining hypoxemia.

The range for oxygen for most of my older patients on day-by-day basis was between 92 and 98. If a person's oxygen level is below 88, then I know that they are deprived of oxygen to the brain and all tissues, and may need supplemental oxygen. Once a person is given supplemental oxygen, they act and look much better. This condition is called hypoxemia or hypoxia.

Some other symptoms of hypoxemia are:

- Changes in the color of the skin from blue to cherry red
- Fast heart rate
- Rapid breathing
- Shortness of breath
- Slow heart rate
- Sweating
- Wheezing

This condition is a medical emergency so call 911.

What conditions cause hypoxemia:

- Asthma attack
- lung diseases such as COPD (emphysema, bronchitis, pneumonia or pulmonary edema)
- Heart problems
- Anemia
- Strong pain medicines and other drugs that change breathing rates

(See "How to care for your Respiratory Equipment" under the first section)

Pain- How do you manage it?

Pain is such a subjective symptom. People are all different in how they tolerate pain. I attended a lecture about pain management a few months ago. I watched the instructor come in the room carrying a blow-up cushion and proceeded to place it on a metal chair left for him to use during the day. He began to tell us that he had had chronic pain all his life from multiple back surgeries, all of which he said he has learned to live with. He says that he would wake up every day and say "hello pain," and proceed with his day. He found that pain was now a part of him, and he could either lie down and not move, or make the best of his day. He knew that even if he moved with the pain, he would not injure himself, and so, that was how he lived his life. Pain is unique to each individual and is a truly personal experience.

First let's talk about acute pain. Acute pain results from a disease, an inflammation (like swelling, redness, heat, and infection), or an injury. Acute pain comes on goes away quickly. Once healing occurs, acute pain is resolved.

Chronic pain is defined as pain that lasts more than 3 months. It starts with an illness or an injury but continues even after healing has occurred because nerves in the tissues have been affected. Because the nerves involved in pain undergo changes that can worsen over time, "chronic pain is now thought to be a disease in itself."

(Institute of Medicine (2011). Relieving Pain in America: A Blueprint for Transforming Prevention, Care, Education, and Research Washington, DC: the National Academies Press.)

According to the CDC, over 51.6 million U.S. adults, or 20.9% of the population, experienced chronic pain in 2021. 17.1 million people, or 6.9% of adults, experienced high-impact chronic pain, which significantly limits daily activities.

Some forms of chronic pain include low back pain, arthritis pain, as well as cancer pain. Headaches, muscle pain, and nerve pain that was once acute and now is persistent can be more sensitive to physical and emotional stresses. This is why pain gets worse when sleep is poor because emotions are linked to this sensation.

Self-management programs are for those who suffer from chronic pain. You can become an active participant by helping with problem-solving, taking action to manage your pain, and learn techniques that could change the way you think and feel about pain.

Pain can be managed a number of ways:

- Over-the-counter remedies
- Prescription medications to relieve pain
- Use of ice, heat, massage, topical creams such as Asper creme
- Stress reduction through relaxation means
- Use of complementary and alternative medicine
- Try soft music, back rubs, a pillow to support the painful area, regular periods of rest from overuse.

I found this cool device called Click Heat. It is a reusable hot or cold pack, which can save you a lot of money if you use disposable ones all of the time. It is a plastic pouch filled with sodium acetate that when a metal disk is flexed, the pack is activated to a temperature of 130 degrees F. You can wrap it in a moist towel and use it up to an hour. To reset it to use it again, just place it in a cloth towel and boil it for 15 minutes. Place it in the fridge, and you have a cool pack. Check it out online: www.clickheat.eu

Chronic pain may need to be treated with surgery or nerve blocks, acupuncture or electrical stimulation. My brother-in-law, Jim, hobbled around for as long as I have known him. With the way he was walking, we thought his hip needed to be replaced. He was evaluated by his HCP who then sent him to an orthopedist and found to have a twisting or torsion of the nerves near Lumbar 4 and 5, and needed a lumbar spinal fusion to relieve the radiating pain down the left leg, which made him limp. Jim is doing much better, and surgery was his answer.

Working in partnership with your HCP to find an effective treatment plan is key. Taking "pain killers" is not the only pathway available to treat chronic pain. Tricyclics antidepressants such as Amitriptyline, and anti-seizure medications used to treat nerve pain, such as gabapentin and Lyrica are two other medications that treat the nerve pathway. Also, SSRIs like Zoloft and norepinephrine reuptake inhibitors (SNRIs) such as Cymbalta, work on another pathway for pain.

Back Pain

Back pain is second to headaches, as reportable pain. A ruptured (herniated) disc or bone spur causes pressure on the spinal nerve radiating pain down a leg and is called "sciatica." Pain in the back could also just be from a muscle spasm. Bed rest is only for an acute episode and should not be done for more than 48 hours. Use of ice wrapped in a towel 30 minutes on, 2 hours off, is very helpful for the first 48 hours, then do the same with heat.

To prevent back problems, remain active. Avoid doing activities which require sudden body movements. Make sure to stretch every day. Swimming and walking are safe exercises to do regularly. Use good posture and avoid gaining excessive weight.

Seek immediate attention if:

- numbness, tingling or weakness of an arm or leg
- Severe back pain not relieved with medications

- Change in bowel or bladder control
- Shortness of breath or dizziness
- Nausea, vomiting or sweats

Everyone has their own pain, so different methods of treatment need to be introduced to determine what it is that needs to be done or changed in your activity to reduce or alleviate pain. Many people do better with their pain if they understand what causes it, what makes the pain worse, and what makes the pain better. Psychotherapy and behavioral modification can help you get control of your pain- which can be very powerful.

Pain management for an older adult need to be handled differently than the younger person. He does not handle the same dosing, so use the motto "start low, go slow" for all medications. In addition, he is taking other medications that can have interactions with other medications. It is important that all medications and supplements are purchased in the same pharmacy so interactions can be found by the pharmacist. When the older person complains of dizziness, weakness or stomach problems, it may not be due to age-related complaints but side effects from some medications.

What should you ask your HCP about your pain?

Asking the following questions can help you understand why you have pain and what you can do to treat it.

- What is causing my pain? What can I do about it?
- Will you or someone else be treating my pain?
- How long will it take for medication to work?
- What are the side effects I should expect, and if I have any, should I call you?
- What should I do if I forget to take the medication?
- What is the proper time of day to take this medication?

- Is there any danger of taking this medication?
- Can I treat my chronic pain without medication?
- What else can I do to manage my pain?

Tracking Your Pain from Visit to Visit:

It is a good idea to formulate a pain diary to keep track of symptoms and its reaction to medicines over a period of time. This way, when you see your HCP or pain management provider, they will have a better understanding of how you are doing and what they can do to help further relieve your pain. Some of the areas you want to address are: the description of your pain, its location, duration, what makes it worse or better, the intensity of it, any other symptoms.

American Chronic Pain Association (www.theacpa.org)

Sometimes people do not want to tell their HCP that they have pain. They may feel the pain is an expected part of their problems, and that they may be thought of as being "weak" or a "complainer." It is important, to be honest. When you have addressed your pain, you can actually improve your quality of life. The HCP will need to know what medications you have tried in the past, both prescriptive and over-the-counter, other treatments including complementary, and what are your goals for pain relief.

Pain medication may be prescribed for the treatment of chronic pain. The health care arena has changed because it has been found that people are asking for medication that is thought to be causing addiction, especially when it comes to opioids. People on hospice (with less than 6 months to live), palliative care, or cancer, not in remission are allowed long-term use of opioids. This new legislation had been introduced as of April 2019 in NY and is now being mandated all over the U.S. There are, however, strict guidelines that have been developed by the CDC to guide your HCP when prescribing opioids. In addition, there is a site called Prescription Drug Monitoring Program

(PDMP) where clinicians can see if a person is getting narcotics from other providers in other states.

What are opioids?

Opioids are narcotics. Examples are: Codeine, Dilaudid, Fentanyl, Oxycontin, Hydrocodone, Morphine and Oxycodone. These medications were initially used for pain due to trauma and acute pain. The side effects are itching, constipation, vomiting, and nausea. They are known to induce sedation as well as relieve pain.

Some people become physically dependent on them. This dependency occurs when opioids are taken for more than 2 weeks' time. A person will experience withdrawal if they stop the medication abruptly. The symptoms are restlessness, muscle and bone pain, insomnia, diarrhea, vomiting, goosebumps, and uncontrollable leg movements.

Tolerance occurs when your body gets accustomed to a medication and you do not get relief pain from the same dose. It is important to talk with your provider before increasing the dose.

An addiction disorder can occur in a small number of people who are taking opioids for pain relief. The person gets "consumed" by the drug, which affects work, home life and other relationships. The drug is being used as a mental stimulant to feel good, but not for any pain relief. The person craves the medication.

Therefore, patients given opioids must be monitored carefully. Opioids have been associated with increased incidents of death when taken with sleep aids, alcohol, and muscle relaxants by slowing breathing then stopping it. Naloxone is a medication given by injection or nasal spray to reverse the effect of the opioid therefore can save a life.

Long-term use of an opioid can change the pain intensity. A clinician will reduce or stop the opioid, give naloxone to reduce the craving for the medication, and recommend the person enter a support group. By doing this, the person can get through his withdrawal.

An important question to ask the person on opioids: What are you able to do now that you were not able to do before taking the medication?

There are other means to try in order to improve chronic pain. Although this type of pain cannot be cured, it can be managed. Here are some methods:

Acetaminophen (Tylenol)

Tylenol, as you know, is an over-the-counter medication. It is also part of over 600 other products. Log onto www.tylenol.com/getreliefresponsibly/home for information about how to use Tylenol safely. Tylenol has been considered the gold standard for relief of pain from osteoarthritis. For adults over 12, the recommended dose is 650 to 1000 mg every 4 to 6 hours, and not to exceed 4,000mg in 24 hours. If you are taking the extended-release version, it is recommended to take 1,300 mg every 8 hours, and not to exceed 3,900 mg in 24 hours. Tylenol can also cause changes in the liver when it is taken at high doses over many years.

Acupuncture

One of the oldest healing modalities from traditional Chinese medicine is the use of needles applied to the skin. This treatment has been known to produce pain relief with no real side effects.

Analgesics

These medications are pain relievers: acetaminophen, ibuprofen as well as opioids. Non-prescription pain relievers treat mild to moderate pain, while prescription pain relievers help with moderate to severe pain.

Anti-anxiety drugs

Valium is a muscle relaxant and is also used for pain relief. It is called a benzodiazepine.

Anti-depressants

Medications such as Zoloft, Celexa and Lexapro are used to treat pain because they can affect mood and thinking patterns.

Anti-migraine drugs

Medications such as Imitrex, Amerge, and Zomig are for treating migraine headaches. They are in class called triptans.

Aspirin

Aspirin is over the counter and is highly used for pain relief. People on blood thinners such as omega 3 fish oil, baby aspirin, and coumadin should avoid taking additional aspirin products as they could cause abnormal bleeding.

Biofeedback

Biofeedback is used to treat mostly headache and back pain. It is an electronic machine that reads muscle tension, heart rate, and skin temperature. It trains you to become aware of these body functions so that you become in control of them to lessen your pain.

Chiropractic

Works with manual therapy by adjusting the spine, which can ease back pain, neck pain, headaches, and musculoskeletal conditions.

Cognitive-Behavioral Therapy (CBT)

Therapy that teaches the person coping skills and relaxation techniques to help manage pain. CBT is used for cancer pain, chronic pain and childbirth.

COX-2 inhibitors

Celebrex is used to treat arthritis. It is a non-steroidal anti-inflammatory (NSAID) similar to Ibuprofen, Naproxen, and Aspirin. They block two enzymes COX-1 and COX-2, which cause inflammation, fever, and pain, while Celebrex only blocks COX-2. Celebrex is less likely to cause stomach ulcers, as opposed to Aspirin and Ibuprofen which can.

Electrical stimulation

TENS (transcutaneous electrical nerve stimulation) is used to stimulate nerves in muscles to help relieve pain.

Exercise

Light to moderate exercise, such as walking and stretching. Exercise contributes to an overall sense of well-being by improving blood and oxygen flow to muscles.

Muscle Relaxants

Cyclobenzaprine (Flexeril) is used to relieve pain and stiffness in muscles and can help with muscle spasms. Use caution if you have an irregular heart rate, glaucoma, overactive thyroid, difficulty urinating, or have heart disease. This medication is not to be taken with medications for mental depression or psychosis.

Physical therapy and rehabilitation

Use of heat, cold, exercise, massage, and manipulation of muscles to treat certain conditions. Techniques such as these help to increase function, control pain and improve recovery especially after surgery.

Surgery

This is the option but is saved as a last resort, especially for back problems.

Resources:

American Academy of Hospice and Palliative Medicine
American Chronic Pain Association
American Headache Society Committee for headache Education
American Pain Society
American Society of Addiction Medicine
Arthritis Foundation
National headache Foundation

Palliative Care-what is it?

Palliative care is specialized medical care for people with a serious illness. The focus of this care is to provide relief from the symptoms and stress of a serious illness. Improving the quality of life for the patient and their family is the goal. Serious illnesses can include cancer, heart disease, lung disease, kidney disease, Alzheimer's disease, ALS, multiple sclerosis, lymphoma, and Parkinson's disease. Most insurances cover Palliative Care.

Palliative care can be provided in a hospital, outpatient clinic and at home. A palliative care team works with other clinicians to provide an "extra layer" of support for you and your family. More time is used for symptom management, communication of your goals, and help with the navigation of the health system. The team also works with treatment meant to cure. Most programs also have hospice programs, so if your mother's condition worsens, she can be moved into the hospice program.

Go to getpalliativecare.org for more information and to find a program near you. Just put in your zip code and see what home programs exist around you.

Parkinson's Disease

This disease is a long-term degenerative disorder of the central nervous system that mainly affects the motor system (which involves movement). Non-motor symptoms, however, become increasingly common as the disease worsens. Symptoms can be a resting tremor, the rigidity of one side of the body, difficulty thinking, and slow movements. This disease involves a deficiency of the neurotransmitter dopamine.

Males ages 50-60 years is the common age of presentation. Depression, fatigue, anxiety and some memory loss can be the first symptoms but are hard to pinpoint with a diagnosis. The needed finding to diagnose Parkinson's disease is bradykinesia- slowness of movement when using hands and legs. A decrease in facial expressions and/or stiffness of the one side of the body are observed.

My very good friends are on their own journey. Here is their story:

Shazam (Sam) was a vibrant, active person preparing for his retirement at the age of 64. One day, while on his daily walk with his wife, he noticed his left arm hanging still by his side while his right arm kept rhythm with his right leg. He also noticed that his left leg was feeling weak. These 2 signs were the beginning of a 4-year journey through a maze of doctors- both medical and holistic- asking hundreds of questions which led to even more questions.

During his quest for answers, he saw 4 different neurologists, all confirming Parkinson's disease. He tried Levodopa/Carbidopa, but the medication made him extremely fatigued. He also complained of brain fog, and after seeing a neuropsychologist and found to have beginnings of Lewy body dementia. He was sent to an Ears, Nose and Throat specialist (ENT) because his voice was changing, and found to have a paralyzed left vocal cord and Lyme disease, of which he was treated with 3 months of antibiotics. He also saw an integrative doctor and was given Meyers Cocktails and glutathione infusions without much help for his fatigue.

Sam looked for ways to help himself as keeping his body as active and healthy as possible. This included following a better diet, fast-walking daily, qigong lessons, and attending Rock Steady Boxing classes. He found a book, "How the Brain Heals Itself" by Dr. Norman Doidge, which has become somewhat of a bible for Sam.

In this book, he learned about a new device coming to the market called the PoNS device from Helius Technologies. It is a non-invasive tongue device which will rewire the brain and bypass damage caused by neurological diseases. It is used to improve gait in the patient with MS or other neurological disorders.

I have also come across an item called the tourmaline-infused blankets. The blankets contain nanoparticles of tourmaline crystals which is permanently adhered to the fabric. This mineral enhances the flow of Qi (energy). The blanket absorbs body heat and re-radiates it into the body as infrared energy. Tourmaline has been known to be beneficial for thousands of years. The blankets can be purchased online.

If you would like to experience movement and exercises by Alex Karten, go to YouTube "Goodbye Parkinson's, Hello Life!" This site talks briefly about his book for Parkinson's patients, and also shows you a demonstration of his 5 components of movement for people with Parkinson's disease to be done every day.

Susan Lust, my colleague, is a certified movement therapist, certified in Gyro-Kinetics. Gyro-Kinetics was founded by Mr. Karten and is a blend of martial arts, structuring and healing movement and music. She is presently working under the preceptorship of Mr. Karten. If you are interested in learning more about the program and perhaps doing Skype sessions for 1:1 training, email SJLust@gmail.com.

Check out "Moving Through Glass"- a Google Glass App, which Mark Morris Dance Group in partnership with SS+K, has created to enable people with PD to use strategies of professional dancers to improve movement, in the comfort of their own home. It is a DVD series that features a menu of visual and musical cueing systems to initiate and support dance moves and fluid, rhythmic walking. It helps people regain a sense of control.

There are 4 modules:

Warm Me Up
Balance Me
Walk With Me
Unfreeze Me
For more information, visit moving through glass.org or email mtg@danceforpd.org

Here are some good reads that I found along the way:
"Goodbye Parkinson's: Hello Life" by Alex Karten
"How the Brain Heals Itself" by Dr. Norman Doidge

Philippians 4:13
I can do all things through him who strengthens me.

Pneumonia

Pneumonia can be detected by someone having an oral low-grade fever of 100.4 degrees F, cough, loss of appetite, and occasional trouble breathing. Sometimes, the person is sleeping more than usual, has a change in their mental status, and/or is just "not right." The lungs may have areas of rales which are crackling sounds not cleared when taking a deep breath or coughing.

A chest x-ray will show opacities or "foggy" looking patches indicating congestion. If the person is dehydrated, pneumonia can be missed on an x-ray. Once the person gets hydrated, the pneumonia is evident. So, if you suspect pneumonia, the person may need to have IV hydration.

Treatment would include an antibiotic, (sometimes a nebulizer with a prescription medication to open the airways), lots of fluids, turning in bed from side to side to move secretions, and a mucolytic such as Robitussin. There is a procedure called cupping and clapping that can mechanically move secretions by cupping your hands. You can also use oxygen face masks to make cupping easier on your hands. This procedure is called chest physiotherapy.

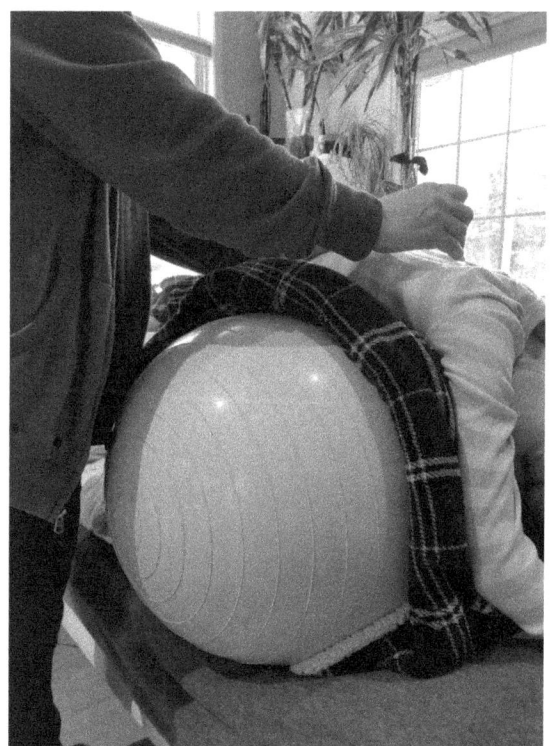 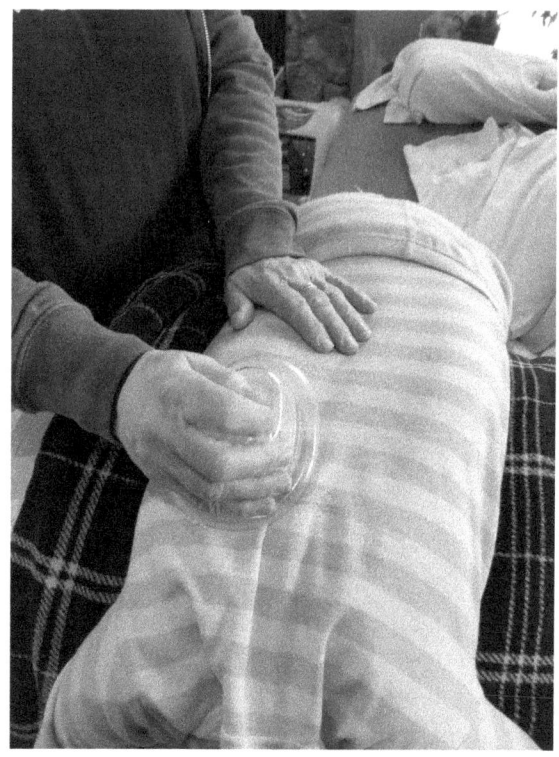

Cupping/chest therapy

Chest physiotherapy is the use of mechanical techniques for clearance of mucus from the airways. By percussing or clapping on the back, you are able to move secretions so the person can cough them up. Sometimes, the use of a suction machine is needed if the person cannot follow your command to "cough it up." This process helps reduce the chance of pneumonia. (Go to Section 1: How to use/care for your portable suction machine).

Using a nebulizer is also great for "respiratory toilet." By using a dilator for the lungs, such as low dose Albuterol three times a day, the person inhales the medicine with the use of the nebulizer and is able to cough and move secretions around. I regularly order a nebulizer for patients who are bedridden and do not move around much.

(Go to the section: How to take care of your nebulizer in Section 1)

Aspiration Pneumonia

This is a good time to discuss aspiration pneumonia. This is congestion in the lungs that occurs when liquids or food "goes down the wrong pipe." People who are bedridden and are fed while lying down or at a 45-degree angle, with a poor swallow reflex, will definitely be at risk for Aspiration Pneumonia. (see Section 2: Aspiration- how to prevent it).

Probiotics- how do they help the gut?

Antibiotics have risks and benefits. The older person is at greater risk of urinary tract infection, skin infections, and pneumonia. If the patient shows any of these problems, whether it is viral or not, an antibiotic is usually prescribed. Sometimes the person continues to have symptoms, even after taking the antibiotic. Either this indicates the "bug and the drug" did not match, or it was just a virus.

Antibiotics can wipe out the normal flora,or good bacteria, in the gut which is needed to control other organisms that reside in the gut, causing another infection called C. *Diff* (Clostridium Difficile). The gut flora is not replenished for almost two years after only one treatment of antibiotics! Diarrhea that is persistent during or after an antibiotic is the first sign that your mother might have this condition. In addition, she might have a fever, loss of appetite, nausea and abdominal pain/tenderness. With a stool test done this organism is found, and oral Vancomycin would then be initiated.

Probiotics fortify digestive health by promoting healthy bacteria. Not all probiotics are the same. When a pill is swallowed and is in the stomach, acid immediately starts to break it down. Live flora such as acidophilus, is eradicated, so the flora is not active any longer. Make sure to find a reputable probiotic that is proven to stay intact until it enters the small intestine.

Probiotic foods include:

- Kefir
- Sauerkraut
- Yogurt
- Pickled cucumber
- Sourdough
- Dark chocolate
- Cottage cheese
- Apple cider vinegar

Restless Legs Syndrome (RLS)

This syndrome is caused by a neurological disorder. It causes the person to feel like the legs cannot stop moving. They may also complain of the jitteriness, itching, burning and tugging of the legs. These sensations have been found to happen in the arms. Symptoms mostly occur when sitting or lying still but improves with activity.

It has been found that the two most common conditions that attribute to RLS is iron malabsorption and nerve damage.

How to limit the symptoms:

- Get a good night's sleep
- Consider taking supplements such as magnesium, folic acid and vitamin B12
- Exercise every day
- Stretch your legs at the beginning and end of each day
- Avoid nicotine, alcohol and caffeine several hours before bedtime

Skin Conditions and Care

Items needed to keep your skin dry and intact:

- Corn starch or non- medicated gold bond powder- your new best friend!
- Cotton strips cut in 8 x6 inches- use white tee shirts, which are washable
- If there are skin folds, moisture will undoubtedly collect in these areas. This is where yeast and fungus love to live because they like it dark and moist. You will see patches of reddened skin, with occasional bleeding and raw skin appearance.
- First, wash the area with soap and water, and dry well by patting the skin. Avoid rubbing this fragile skin to prevent opening wounds.
- Place a little bit of powder in gloved hands and clap your hands lightly to remove excess.
- Pat powdered hands under breasts, armpits and between skin folds. (The reason to use light powder and not to shake the bottle on the skin is to avoid a pastry- like excess of the powder which is hard to remove.)

Preventing Skin Tears

As we age, the skin on the arms and legs gets thinner causing easy black and blues, bruises, and the worst is skin tears. If you notice dark bruises on the arms or legs, which sometimes, has no history of trauma, it is time to protect the skin. Also, being on any kind of blood thinners like Eliquis puts the older person more at risk for skin tears.

I like to use items that are washable and already around the house. All you need is a soft pair of socks- better if men's white sport socks. Some women

SKIN CONDITIONS AND CARE

may not find this fashionable so get creative! Get colorful socks as long as they are soft, loose and made of cotton.

Even if the person wears sweat pants, put the socks on the legs for protection after daily washing. On the arms, just cut off the toe part, turn the sock around, so the cuff that is usually at the knee is at the wrist area, and the heel now fits on the elbow. If the hands have ecchymoses (bruises), you can cut a hole in the sock about one inch up and slide the thumb in. Now the hand is protected too.

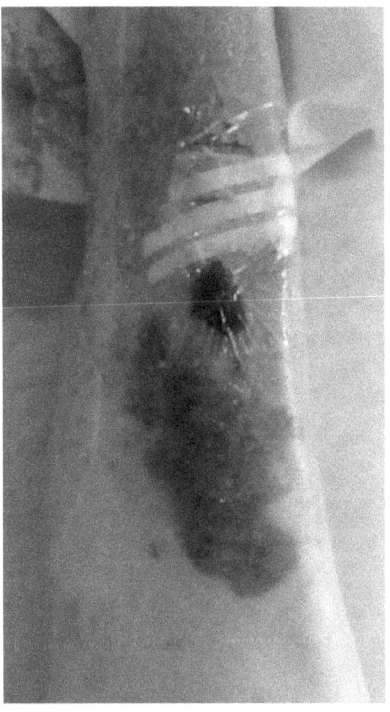

This is why you wear a protective sock

Skin tears occur when the bruises get injured peeling back the top layer of the skin like a window shade rolled up. When this happens, it is best to see if you can unravel the skin to replace it over the new open area. Once the skin is removed, you lost the protective layer on the surface of the skin (the epidermis). The wound has a bigger chance of infection and poor healing.

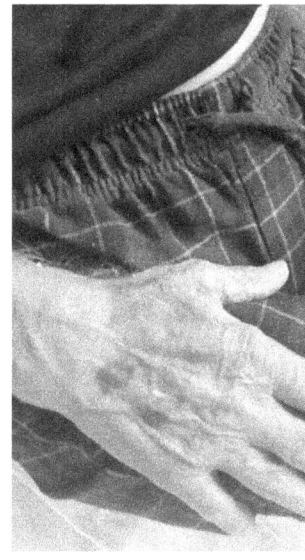
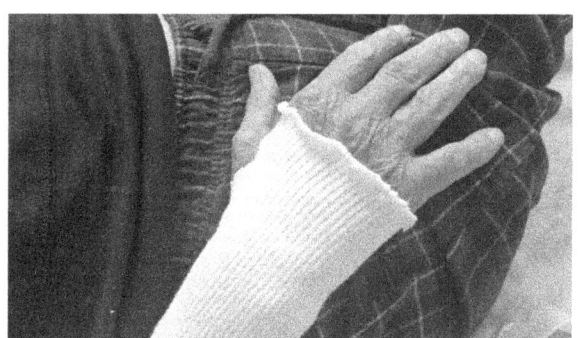
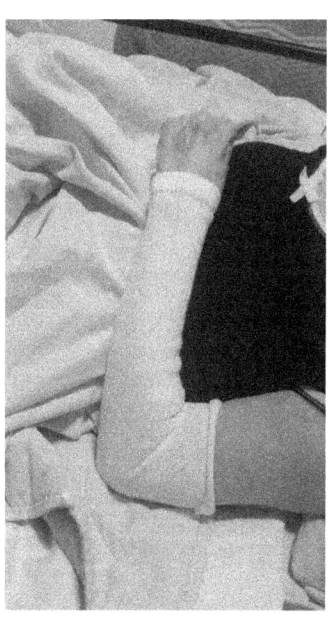

Also, it is good to know if the person had a tetanus shot in the last 10 years- now getting the Tdap which includes tetanus toxoid and acellular pertussis. This is a vaccine that you can get from your HCP.

If you get a skin tear these are items needed (get all items from the pharmacy or local grocery store):

- Saline for washing the wound (wound wash in a can)
- Vinyl gloves
- Package of non- sterile 4 x 4 gauze pads
- Steri-strips - 1/8 inch
- Non-stick pads without adhesive
- Kling wrap (gauze)
- Tape

Instructions to care for a skin tear:

- Wash your hands thoroughly and don a pair of gloves
- Spray saline on the skin tear
- If the skin is rolled up, gently try to unravel the skin using saline to keep it moist. Even if only some of the skin remains, flatten it out and cover the open wound with it.
- Once the skin is intact, gently pat it dry with a gauze pad
- Cut the steri-strips in 1/2 or enough to cover the wound and its corners
- Place the strips in a crisscross pattern on top of one another
- Place the non-stick pad on top of the steri-strips
- Wrap the arm (or leg) loosely with Kling wrap - never put the gauze on tight and move the gauze wrap around the leg without overlapping. Do it a few times then cut the Kling and apply a small piece of tape to the Kling.
- Never apply tape around the whole extremity to prevent a tourniquet effect
- Keep the area clean and dry, changing the non-stick dressing and Kling every day for about a week
- The steri-strips stay on for 7 days and may be soiled a little with blood

- Gently remove the top one first, and so on. If you get to the lower steri-strips and the skin does not look intact, then reinforce with a few more steri-strips, and re-bandage it.
- Remove the strips within 10 days and apply a Band-Aid.
- Use the cut-up socks for now on, for good skin protection.

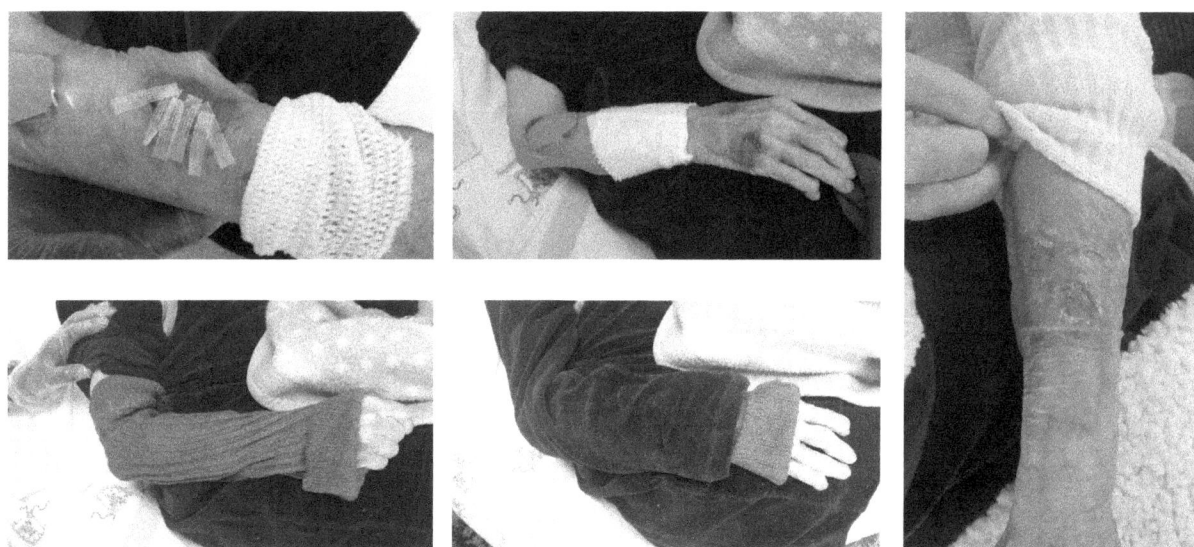

Healed skin tear

Skin Breakdowns: How does a pressure ulcer occur?

Pressure ulcers cause a great burden on the caregiver, the patient who is experiencing them and the general health care system. As of January 2024, the US has a reported prevalence of 2.5 million pressure ulcers. The most anatomical locations for pressure ulcers are the heels and the sacrococcygeal region. The major population at risk are older adults who have multiple risk factors that increase their vulnerability, people who are critically ill and those with spinal cord injury/ disease.

According to an overview that was generated across the web with AI, the cost of caring for a single person with a pressure ulcer can range from $20.900 - $151,700! What is worse, most ulcers could be prevented.

Some of the burdens from bedsores:

- Time and earnings potentially lost from work
- The financial and emotional impact on patient's families
- Forced early retirement for younger patients
- Other expenses associated with morbidity and mortality

What is a pressure ulcer? A pressure ulcer is an injury to the skin and /or underlying tissue usually over an area of the skin where the bone is protruding. When an immobile patient is on his side all of the time, and not turned, a pressure ulcer is sure to happen. It can also happen if sitting in a chair for too long.

A pressure ulcer on the bony part of the spine or other areas can happen because of the bony protrusion causing pressure and the person sat all day without pressure-relieving devices. Another way to have a skin eruption is with "shearing." Shearing is when a body is moved across an area, actually rubbing along, especially while transferring the person to a chair or pulling the person up in bed.

The areas most affected are the hip bones, lower back near the coccyx, elbows, ankles, and even the back of the head or the ear. Any place where a person lies for an indefinite period of time is bound to get a pressure sore (or bedsore).

Braden Risk Assessment Scale

Google the "Braden Scale" developed back in 1988, which remains an effective tool by scoring the person for their risk of developing a pressure ulcer based on 6 factors: sensory perception, moisture, activity, mobility, nutrition and friction/shear. If the person has a score of less than 16, the risk is high for developing a pressure sore.

The higher the risk, the lower the score: 15-18: MILD RISK; 13-14: MODERATE RISK; 10-12: HIGH RISK; < 9: SEVERE RISK. As the person's condition changes, it is a good idea to re-score the person. Not that you should let your guard down at any time because following these measures, you can help reduce skin breakdowns. (Google Braden Risk Assessment Scale to download a copy)

SKIN CONDITIONS AND CARE

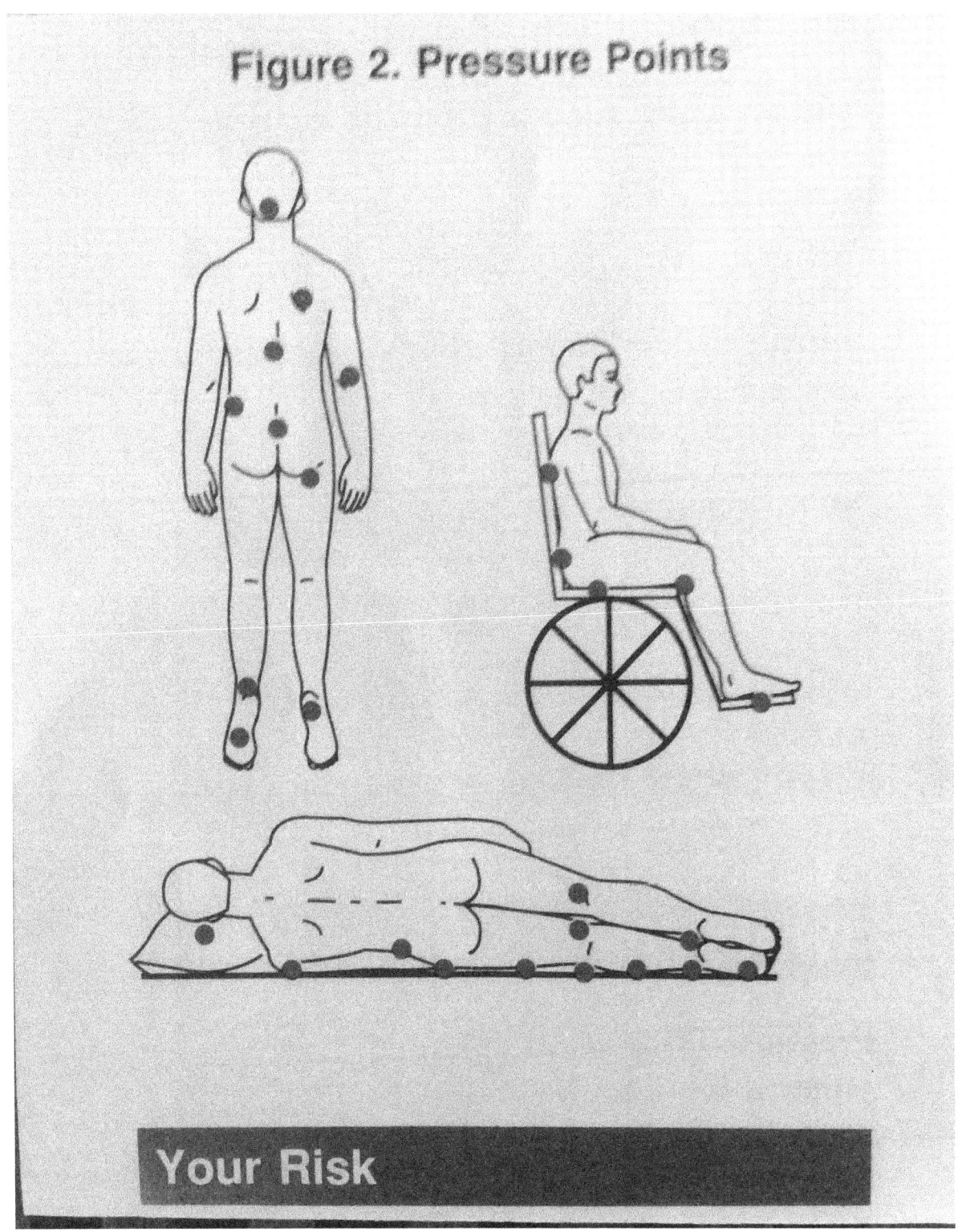

Figure 2. Pressure Points

Your Risk

Here are some risk factors for pressure ulcers:

Lack of movement

When a person lies in the same position for hours, the pressure on the skin reduces blood supply to that area. The picture of the pressure sore on the heel of one of my patients was caused by this (see picture on the next page). She had a stroke and was paralyzed on the right side. She lacked the sensation in her right leg due to this paralysis. You and I would shift in bed if we get uncomfortable; but not so for the weak person. The first sign of injury is that the area looks bruised or very red. The skin is intact, but this can fool you. Through the deep layers of the skin could be where the injury lies. The important thing to know is DO NOT RUB THE SKIN. Doing so can lead to more injury. Moving off of the area, keeping it clean and dry and protecting it with a barrier cream like Balmex will prevent further damage.

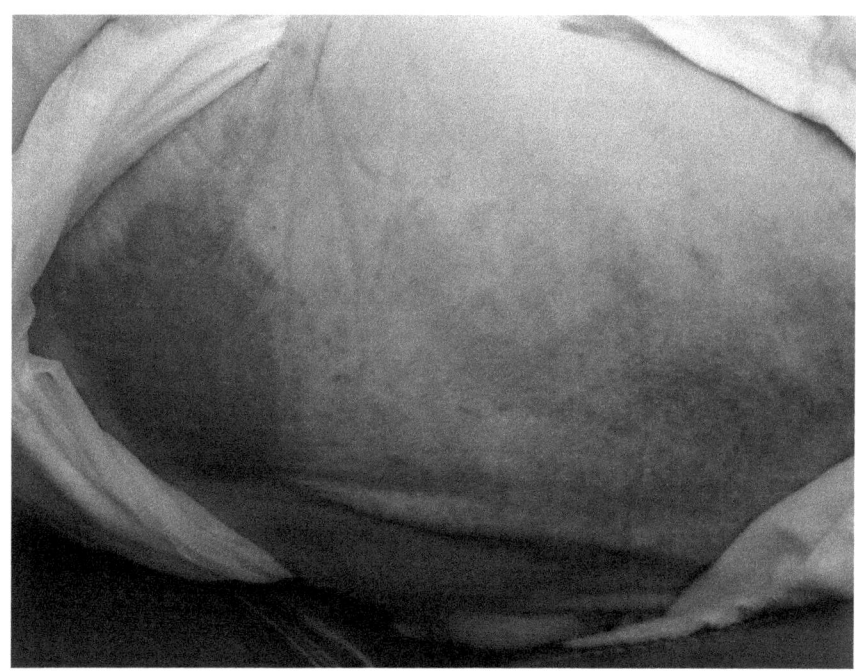

Poor hygiene

A person who is bedridden, or is unable to perform their own personal care, even if mobile, are at risk for skin rashes, and breakdowns. Skin that is very dry and flaking, pimples, odor and rashes in the creases: These are tell-tale signs that the person has not been washing on a regular basis. Sometimes you can see brown crusty patches from lack of washing.

Urinary incontinence (unable to hold urine), and other sources of moisture

Proper cleaning of the perineal area using soap and water, or baby wipes with period under garment changes, are necessary. The longer urine sits on the skin, the more chances of skin breakdown. Having a colostomy that is leaking under the colostomy barrier called a wafer, is also a source of moisture and can lead to skin eruptions.

Diabetes and other sources of poor circulation

Diabetes is a culprit for altering circulation, therefore, it affects the skin as well. Keeping blood sugar under control is necessary to reduce skin injury.

Peripheral Vascular Disease

The way to tell if there are circulation changes of the lower legs, for instance, is the change in the skin color. Usually, it has a brownish patchy or "knee sock" appearance. The skin is susceptible to bruising and can wounds can be difficult to heal. The older skin becomes less elastic and wrinkled. Getting an injury on this area can lead to big problems for the person. It is very important to protect the skin from injury at all times: long cotton socks, sweat pants, flannel clothing, layering, and don't forget the slippers to protect the feet!

Venous ulcers are the most common type of leg wound due to abnormal valve function. The wound cannot heal with edema present. The wound appears on the lower leg, are shallow, irregularly shaped with a moderate amount of yellow fibrous tissue. Treatment includes wound care and compression therapy.

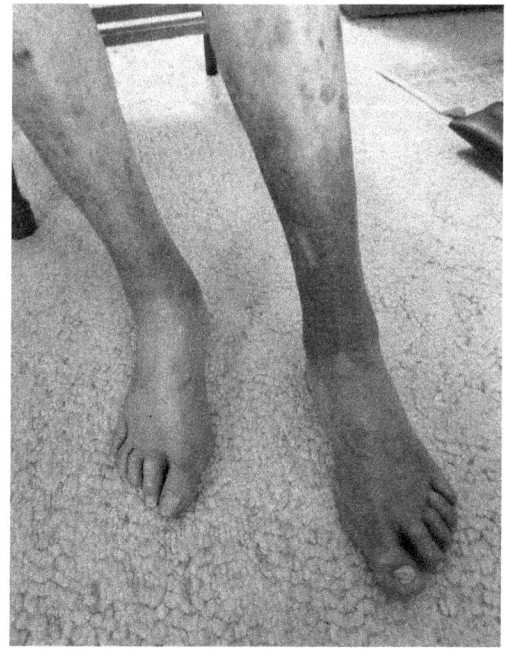

Discolored skin and an open wound

Smoking

Healing of any wound is difficult for a smoker. With every puff of the cigarette, the circulation is diminished causing slow or poor healing.

Being underweight

A thin person will have more bony prominences that cause pressure. Therefore, he is at increased risk for skin injury.

Localized infection or trauma

Cellulitis, contusions, and hematomas are examples of trauma that could lead to pressure ulcers.

Edema (swollen legs or feet due to water retention)

Edema is caused by a collection of fluid under the skin. If it is pitting edema, you can push in the skin with your finger and see a finger imprint. Non-pitting means you cannot produce a dent when the skin is pressed. Compression stockings such as TEDs or ACE wraps can be applied to the legs to help reduce edema.

It is best to apply them before the person comes out of the bed since the swelling is minimized when lying down, and the legs have not been dependent yet. Start at the foot and give the ACE (4 inch is best) gently spiraling it in a crisscross fashion up the leg. Use bandage tape to hold it in place. Never wrap the tape around the leg to prevent a tourniquet effect.

I came across TUBIGRIP at one of my patient's homes. They are elasticized tubular bandages that come in a roll and can be cut and disposed of if soiled. The beauty of them is there is no foot part to fight with and is cut to the length of the sole of the foot up to the knee.

(See pictures of Ace Wrap application and Tubigrip under DVT- What is it and how to prevent it?)

Poor hydration and/or nutrition

For healthy skin, we need to have a healthy diet and drink plenty of fluids. Measuring the albumin and protein in the blood is one factor that indicates whether the diet is healthy. Protein are the building blocks for skin tissue. Most older patients tend to have a low protein level, which puts them at risk for skin breakdown. Eggs, chicken, chickpeas are some examples of high protein foods that can help increase albumin.

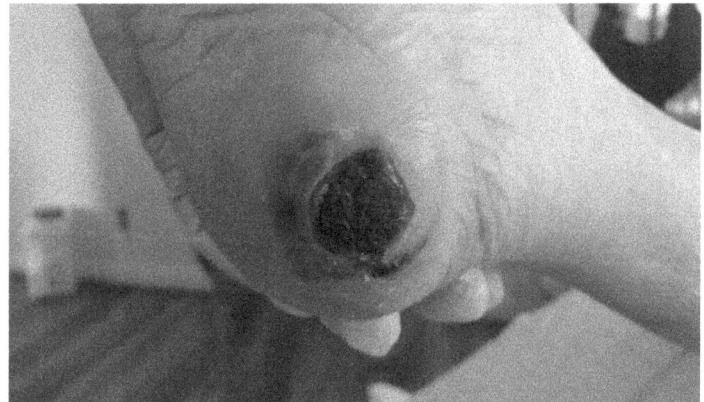

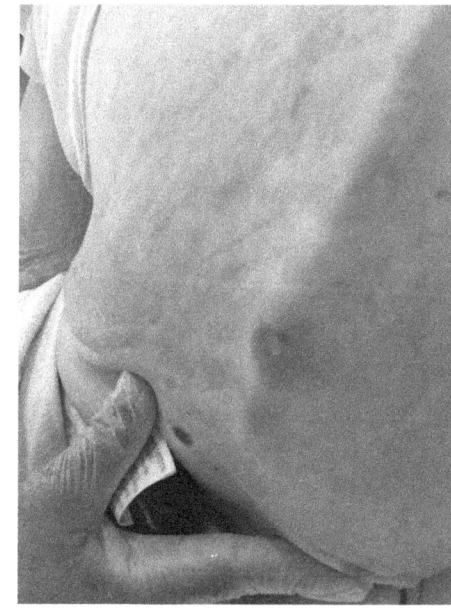

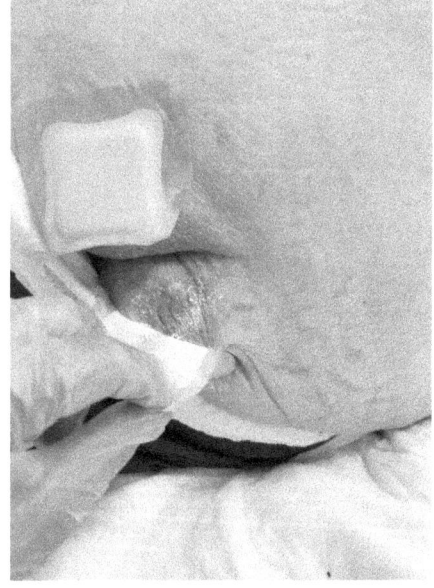

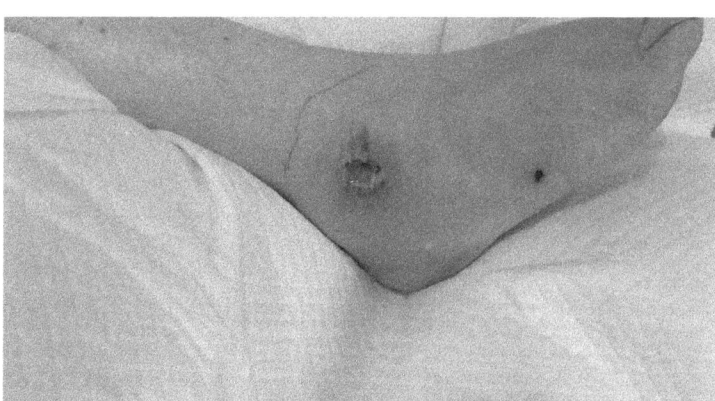

So how do you prevent pressure ulcers?

- Keep the person clean (regular sponge baths with warm water, or better yet, have her sit on a tub transfer seat in the shower for a thorough cleaning. Our skin becomes drier and more damages more easily as we

age. Keeping the skin moisturized after a bath while the skin is slightly damp is crucial for maintaining intact skin.
- Check the person's skin daily for any signs of breakdown or redness
- She should eat plenty of healthy foods, and drink 6 glasses of liquids/day
- Have your mother go to the bathroom every 2- 3 hour to control urination and bowel movements.
- Position her in the bed to alleviate any pressure on bony areas.
- The person should be positioned so there is no pressure on the heels, elbows, head or ears.
- If the person is incontinent, change the undergarment every two hours when in bed and every hour when in a chair.
- Clean her skin well and use a skin barrier cream like Calmoseptine or Balmex
- For an incontinent male, you can add a maxi pad in the front of the undergarment to act as a wick for urine; it can easily be removed and changed
- A gel hybrid seat cushion should be placed on the wheelchair. It can be purchased from the vendor got the wheelchair from.
- Use pillows, foam padding or wedges to keep the person in a good position
- Have your HCP order a gel foam overlay for the mattress, and consider getting a semi-electric hospital bed to make positioning easier for the caregiver.
- Use a folded-up bedsheet in the shape of a square that is placed under the person. This is called a draw sheet. With two people, you can prevent shearing by pulling the person up in bed with the sheet. A trapeze bar can be attached to the hospital bed if the person is strong enough to help pull herself up.
- Keep the head of the bed elevated 30 degrees and the knee gatch up slightly in order to prevent sliding down in bed.

- Keep muscles active by having her move her limbs periodically
- Never massage her calves because it could dislodge a clot.
- DO NOT rub reddened areas on bony areas.
- Vitamin C 500mg /day can help reduce pressure ulcers by providing the skin with an important vitamin
- Position heels over a bolster pillow suspended off of the bed and use a bed board to prevent foot drop

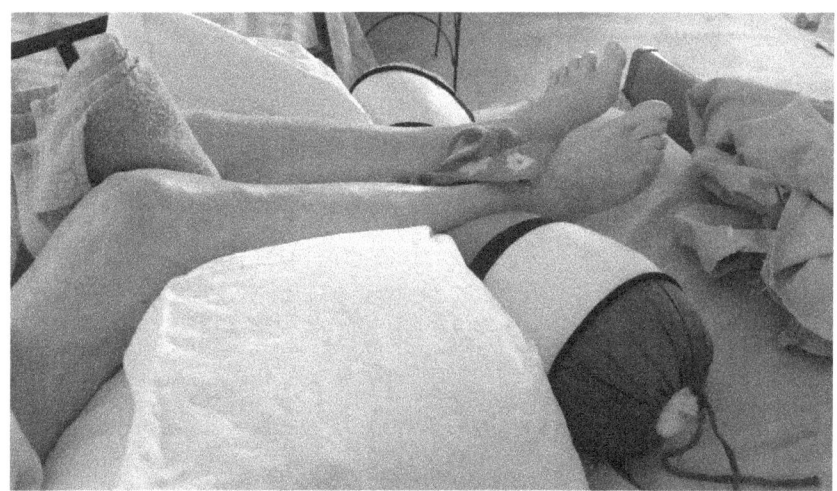

How do you position someone in bed?

- You will need: 2-3 soft pillows
- Always tell the person what you are going to do
- If the person is in a hospital bed, you stand on one side of the bed and lower the bed railing
- Have the person turn to the side opposite you and hold onto the railing
- Help them bend the top leg over, if able, and gently push them over to the side
- Have a folded pillow ready, and place it under the draw sheet near the upper back

SKIN CONDITIONS AND CARE

- Apply a soft pillow between the knees
- Elevate the head of the bed 30 degrees
- Adjust the knee gatch to prevent sliding down
- Check the person for comfort
- Raise the bed railing

Note the time and be ready to turn in the next 2 hours
(Go to YouTube Caregiver Success- How to position a person in bed)

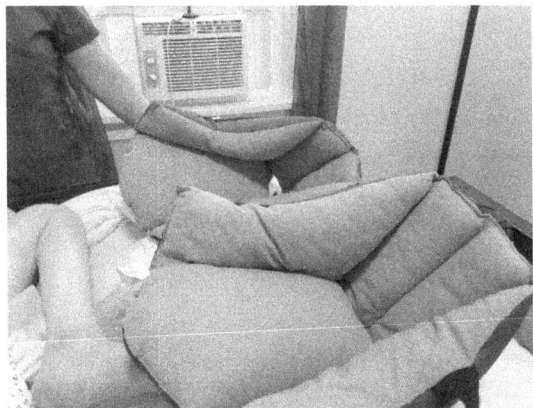
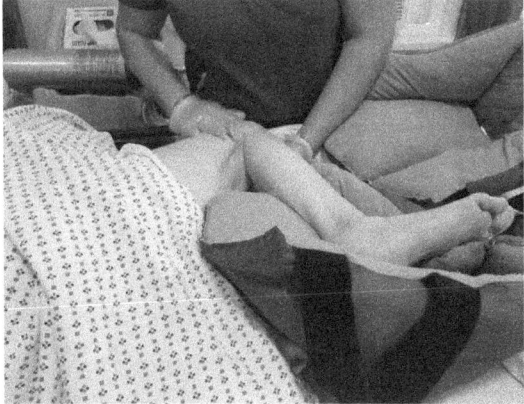

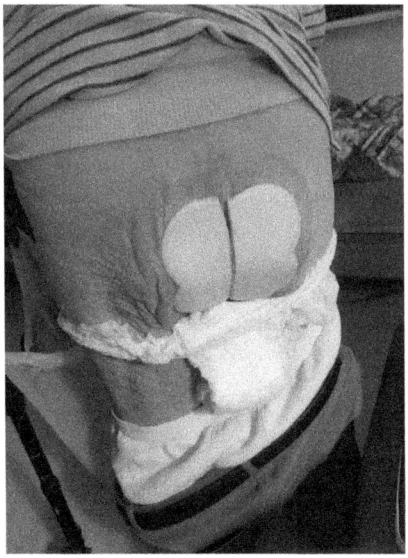

Protection for bony buttocks

How do you know if the wound is infected?

You know when you get a cut in your finger, and it swells, is tender to touch, gets red and warm? Sometimes, there is a thick yellow discharge, or it is green and smells? These are all signs of infection. Sometimes, an antibiotic such as Keflex or Clindamycin needs to be ordered. If so, be sure to start a probiotic with it! This is because antibiotics are known to wipe out your good gut flora and probiotics will help combat this.

There are four stages of Bed Sores (Pressure Ulcers):

It is good to know the stages as the visiting nurse will be talking with you about this. The top layer of our skin is the epidermis; the second layer is called the dermis. This layer is thicker than the epidermis. Stage 3 involves the entire depth of the dermis and now exposes the fat layer but no exposure to bone or tendon. Stage 4 wound involves all the layers of the skin with exposure of bone, muscle or tendon.

Stage 1: skin is intact and not blanchable-meaning when pressed, it does not change a lighter color. This means the circulation of the skin has been impaired. Stage 1 wounds are hard to see when looking at a dark person's skin. It can be cooler than the surrounding skin.

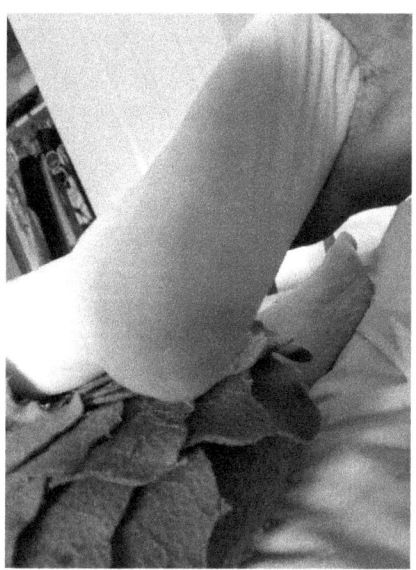

Stage 1 pressure wound

Stage 2: Shallow open ulcer with some loss of the second layer of the skin called the dermis. The wound bed is red-pink and could have a fragile fluid-filled blister.

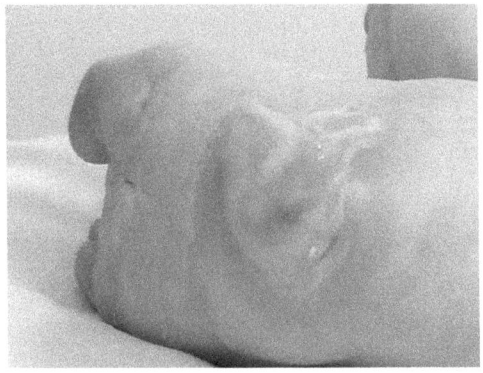

Stage 2 pressure wound

Stage 3: Wound can appear deep as its tissue is lost through the subcutaneous fat layer, but no bone, tendon or muscle is exposed. Tunneling can occur in this stage where the nurse is able to insert a cotton tip applicator into an opening inside of the wound.

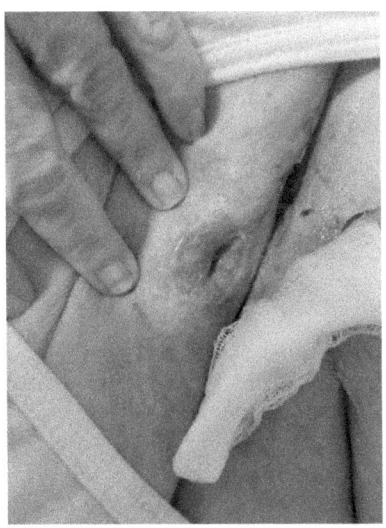

Stage 3 pressure wound

Stage 4: This wound is open through the fat layer and exposes bone, tendon or muscle. This is the worst kind showing a sloughy tissue, some black eschar (dead), tunneling. So, areas such as the buttocks have more fat than the nose so will look to be a deeper wound than a stage 4 wound on the nose. When the bone is involved, this is called osteomyelitis. These wounds can take months to years to heal.

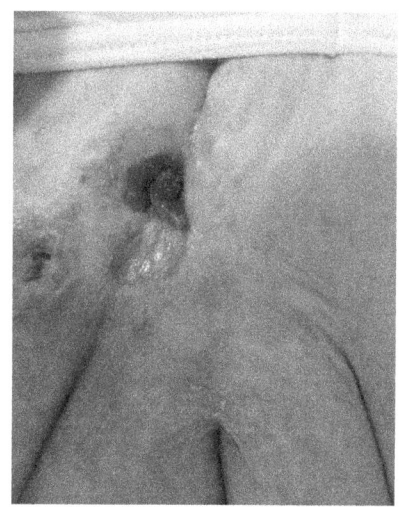

Stage 4 pressure wound

Deep tissue Injury: Purple or maroon area of intact skin or blood-filled blister due to damage of underlying soft tissue from pressure and/or shearing. May show black eschar and may change into a deep ulcer.

Unstageable pressure ulcer: the base of the ulcer is covered with yellow, tan, grey, green or brown slough or eschar which is tan, brown or black. Until the slough is removed and the wound bed is exposed, the depth of the wound cannot be determined.

(www.npuap.org)

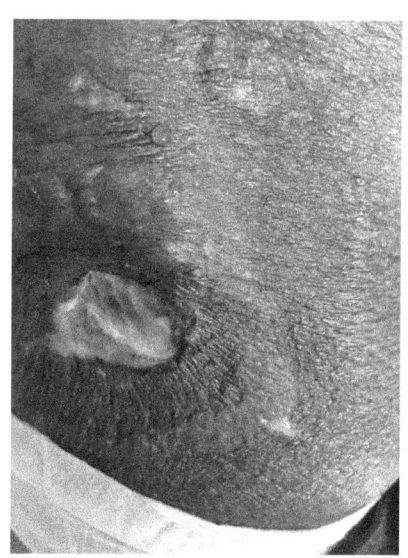

Unstageable wound

Methods used to treat pressure ulcers:

A high-density foam mattress can reduce the chance of new pressure ulcers from occurring by 60%. Sheepskin overlays on top of mattresses were also found to prevent new pressure ulcer formation. (Cochran's Review 2015).

If the wound is necrotic, use of betadine helps to dry the area. Necrotic tissue is dead, non-functioning tissue that cannot use oxygen or nutrients to function normally. The reason for the dead tissue and slough to be removed is to aid in the healing of the wound through all thicknesses. Other areas of the body that have necrotic tissue recommends "debridement" or removal. Collagenase (Santyl) ointment is a product that is made up of enzymes that promote the removal of necrotic tissue. A "wet to dry" dressing is where saline is placed on the wound then a dry dressing. Every day as the dressing is removed, the debris on the wound is gently removed or debrided. This type of wound care is called mechanical debridement.

It is important to have home care nurses, and the wound nurse called to the home for complete guidance, and for dressing supplies through Medicare Part B. When the nurse first assesses the wound, he/she will measure length, width, and depth. As the visits progress, the wound continues to be measured to evaluate the effectiveness of the treatment plan. The depth of the wound is measured using a sterile Q tip. Family members (if available) are taught how to change the dressing. With orders signed by your HCP, this service can be initiated. Call your local Office of the Aging for certified home health agencies near you.

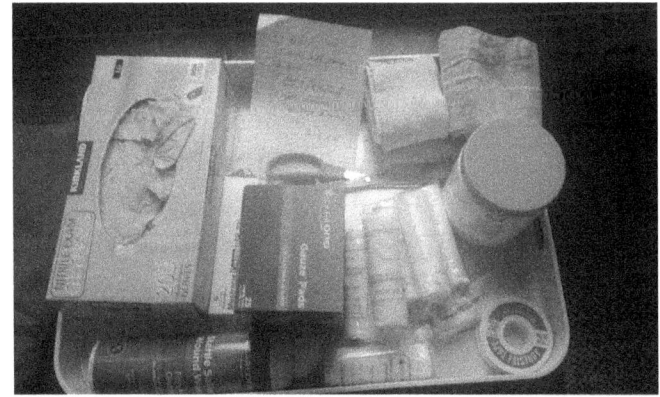

Get organized and keep supplies together

Skin Conditions

Did you know your skin is the largest organ of our bodies? It regulates our temperature with shivering when we are cold, and sweating through our pores when we are hot. It protects our bones and other organs. The nails are also considered a part of our skin.

Let's talk about signs of skin cancer and melanoma, and who is at risk:

Anyone, black or white, can get skin cancer, and if caught early, it is highly treatable.

Every mole, freckle, or age spot has the potential to become cancerous. It is good to have someone look at your back, scalp, behind your ears, lower back, backs of legs, bottom of feet and between toes; which are places you cannot see for skin changes. Sometimes the lesion might be bleeding or is itchy- these are reasons to seek an exam from a dermatologist.

The medical history that you have experienced can increase the risk of getting skin cancer. If you have had blistering sunburns as a child, used indoor tanning devices, been badly burned from an accident or sun, a weakened immune system, or had an organ transplant, you are at risk for skin cancer.

Basal Cell Carcinoma (BCC)

This is the most common type of skin cancer. People at risk are fair- skinned, who freckle easily, red-headed, or light-colored eyes, male and over the age of 50. It takes years for this cancer to develop. This cancer appears in many shapes and sizes. Sometimes the lesions are pearly dome-shaped moles; they can be shiny or scaly, can heal and then return. BCC first develops on the skin that is most exposure from the sun: the scalp, neck, nose, face, and hands. If BCC is not treated, the lesion grows deeper into the skin and damages surrounding tissue, including muscle, bone, and cartilage.

Squamous Cell Carcinoma (SCC)

This type of cancer is the second most common type. It takes many shapes: it can be a bump that bleeds, or a crusted or flat red patch, or a sore that just does not heal. It mostly involves areas of the face, ears, lips, back of hands, legs, and arms. SCC can occur in the mouth and on the genitals (penis or vagina). SCC if not treated, can lead to other areas of the body and then, becomes difficult to treat. Smoking or tobacco chewing may also increase the risk of SCC.

Melanoma

Melanomas can occur anywhere on the body. It can also form in the eyes. Again, exposure to UV light is the cause, as well as involving women under the age of 40. They appear as a new, unusual growth or a change in an existing mole. The mole diameter becomes bigger, with different colors, and irregular borders. Melanoma can be treated successfully if it is found early.

There is a great mnemonic to help you remember what to look for when examining your skin to determine if you have melanoma, the worst form of skin cancer: **A-B-C-D-E**. Any person with any color skin is at risk for melanoma. It can appear on the soles of the feet, under a nail, in the mouth, genitalia, and palms of the hands. The mole under the nail looks like a brown or black streak. A mole that is a melanoma is usually itchy and bleeds.

A-Asymmetry

When you look at a mole or discoloration, imagine putting a line down the middle- does each side look the same? If not, then this is called asymmetry.

B- Border
Look at the edges of the mole- is it jagged, or irregular in shape?

C- Color
Is there more than one color in the lesion- gray, black, red, brown, white or blue?

D- Diameter
Is the colored area bigger than the tip of a pencil eraser?

E- Evolution
A mole that you noticed is changing fast.

If any of these signs occur, it is important to see a dermatologist for a full body exam and any necessary treatment. It may involve a biopsy which will determine the type of skin cancer. People who get skin cancer are prone to getting skin cancer again.

How to examine your skin or someone else's:

- It is good to look at your skin in a full-length mirror in a well-lit room
- Stand in your underwear, or the person fully exposed in bed

Do the following to you and /or the patient:

- Bend elbows and look at forearms, palms of hands and back and upper arms
- Look at feet, soles and between the toes
- Check the back of the neck, scalp by parting the hair and use a hand mirror to help you
- Check back, and buttocks using a hand mirror

How to prevent skin cancer:

- Avoid the sun between the hours of 10 and 2 PM
- Wear sunscreen on all areas of the skin, even on cloudy days
- Wear protective clothing, hats, long-sleeved shirts, sunglasses
- Apply sunscreen that protects your skin from UVA and UVB rays with a (Sun Protection Factor) SPF of at least 30
- Perform skin self-exams
- Take extra sun care around areas of water, snow, and sand as they reflect the sun's rays

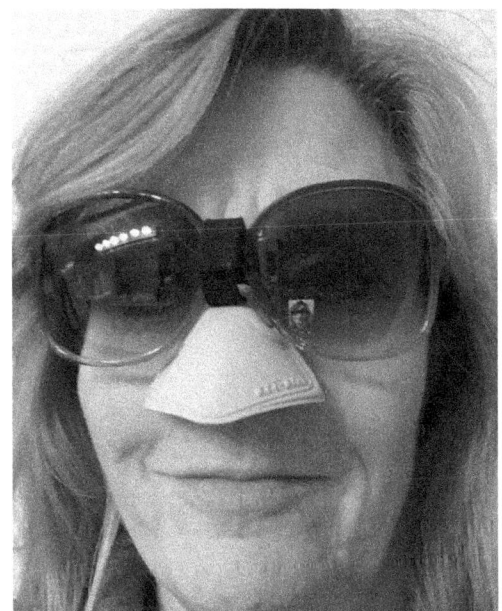

Actinic Keratosis (AK)

This type of skin growth is common but considered precancerous, and if left untreated can lead to SCC. AK can appear as dry, scaly spots on the skin, especially the head, ears, lips, scalp, arms, and hands. They can disappear and then return.

Seborrheic Keratoses (SK)

When I looked at my father, I did inherit his long eyelashes, but I also inherited skin growths from him. One is seborrheic keratosis, of which were multiple scattered brown or tan spots that appear as freckles but have a wart-like texture as if you could remove them with a fingernail. They are considered benign (non-cancerous), but to me, are most irritating and ugly. I found them mostly on my face, neck, chest, and shoulders- right where people look at you. Strawberry warts or hemangiomas are those tiny pinpoint bright red spots that appear any place on the skin. My Dad had a bunch of those too!

Lucky for me, I found a wonderful dermatologist, who every year, would freeze them off- a procedure called cryosurgery, just so I could see him in a year to do it all over again!

(American Academy of Dermatology 1 888-462-3376 or SpotSkinCancer.org)

Let's review types of trauma or infections of the skin:

One important fact is that you should not use hydrogen peroxide or alcohol to clean a wound, as these agents can cause slow healing. Soap from a dispenser and water are the best cleansing agents.

Cellulitis

Cellulitis is a reddened, tender, warm area on the skin. Trauma, such as a laceration (or cut) on the arm can get infected, and spread to a bony area nearby. Bacteria such as staphylococcus or streptococcus can get into the wound. You may see red streaks coming down from the infected site and the person may have an elevated temperature. These symptoms can lead to hospitalization so that intravenous antibiotics need to be started. If the person becomes lethargic or drowsy, has vomiting, diarrhea or generalized weakness with muscle aches, seek medical attention right away.

Also, if a joint nearby becomes painful after the skin has healed, it may mean the cellulitis has returned and would require intravenous antibiotics again. Watch for the development of a boil or swollen bump which may be an abscess. This area would need to have warm moist compresses to help it reach a "head" so it breaks and then drain.

Cellulitis is treated with antibiotics, limb elevation and application of a warm cloth to the area several times a day. If there is a laceration of the skin, it is important to keep it clean and dry. Use saline wound wash and topical antibiotic creams such as Neosporin or bacitracin. Bactroban is a stronger anti-microbial and is used with extremely infected wounds. To prevent recurrence of cellulitis, avoid scrapes or cuts in the skin.

Contusions

A contusion is an area of tenderness and swelling in the soft tissues. It appears as a patch of redness and may bleed. A contusion is caused by damage to the skin, such as banging someone's foot with an object such as a table leg.

What to do:

- Rest the injured area to reduce any pain
- Apply an ice pack or a bag of frozen peas wrapped in a moist towel every few hours for 2 to 3 days
- On day 4, use moist heat for comfort (do not leave it unattended and make sure it is not too hot to prevent burning)
- Compression bandages work well to reduce pain, motion, and swelling

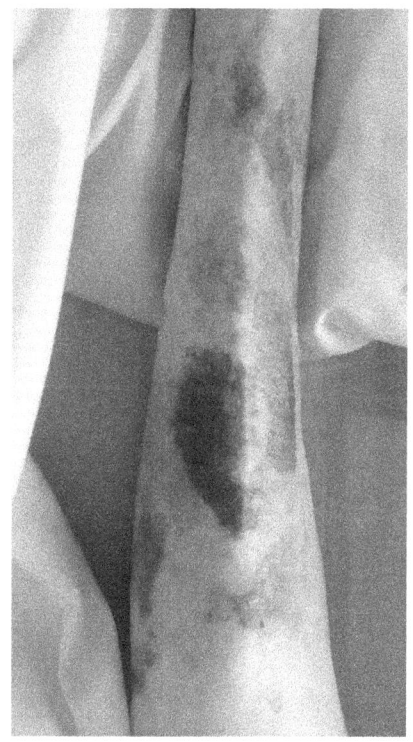

Leg contusion

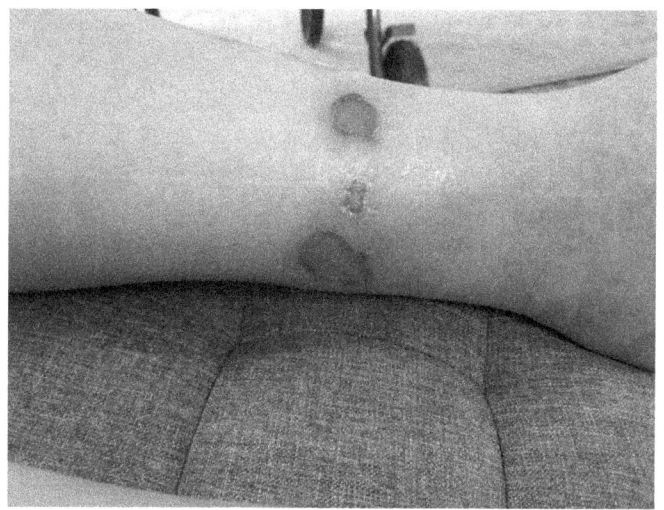

Wound from using tape on skin

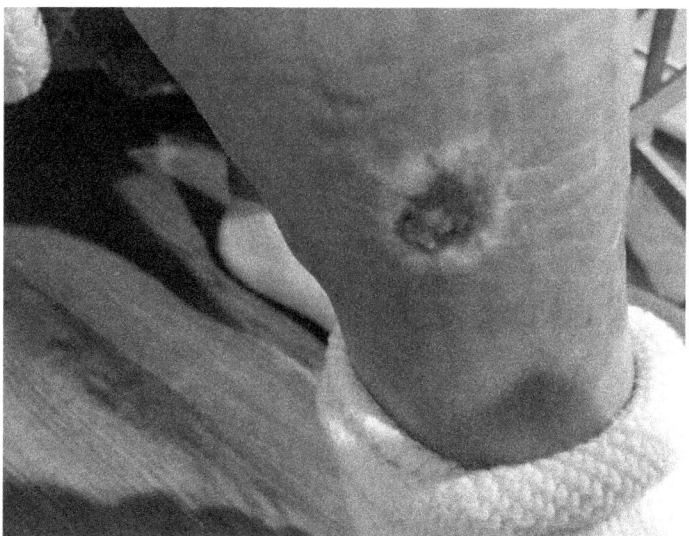

White area around wound is macerated

Folliculitis

Folliculitis is a bacterial infection involving a hair follicle. The area becomes red and irritated. This skin condition occurs on the scalp, thighs, legs, back, and buttocks. It is also found in areas of frequent shaving. When the infection of the follicle goes deeper, it becomes a boil or furuncle. A group of these boils creates something called a carbuncle. A hairy, sweaty area is where they most likely will occur.

How is folliculitis treated?

- Tea tree oil is a great topical antiseptic, which can be found at a health food store.
- Apply a warm compress to the boil three times a day
- If the boil gets a pus head, it can be gently drained
- Personal hygiene using antiseptic washes may help with recurrences

People with long-lasting folliculitis need to find out where the infection is coming from. Germs responsible can live in the nostrils of the patient and can cause an outbreak now and then. The responsible party may be a family member. A topical antibiotic cream such as Bactroban (mupirocin) applied to the inside of the nose twice a day for a week for the patient, but also the family member, then repeated every 6 months is the way to reduce recurrence. Call your HCP if the person has an oral temperature above 100.4 F, or treatment is not improving.

Hematoma

A hematoma is a larger collection of blood that may form in deep tissue (blood blister). It is reabsorbed by the body naturally. Sometimes it needs to be drained. Call your HCP if there are signs of infection (increased redness, swelling, or pain) or numbness or coldness to the injured area.

Herpes Zoster (Shingles)

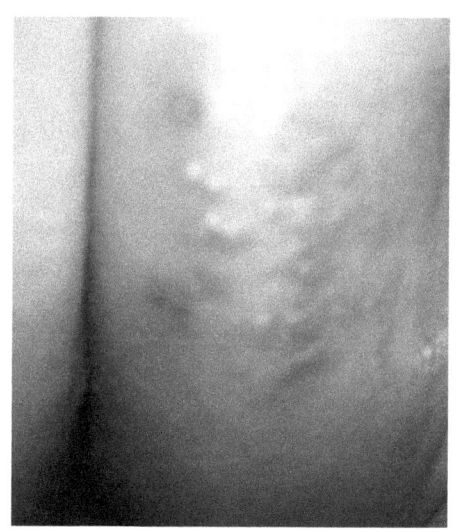

Herpes Zoster, also known as shingles, is identified by blisters, in clusters, and on only one side of the body. Many of us had chicken pox as young children. Throughout the years, chicken pox lays dormant and waits for the opportunity to erupt. Usually, people with low immune systems due to stress, disease, and age, cause this eruption on the skin.

The first symptom is burning and itching with no evidence of a rash. The condition can be mild or severe. The interesting fact is that our bodies have a mapping of something called dermatomes all over us. These dermatomes carry nerve pathways, where the chickenpox lay dormant. Shingles is a blistery rash and has a unique appearance where it does not cross the midline, like drawing a line down the center.

If a blistery rash appears on the face, it is a medical emergency because it can involve the cranial nerves that innervate our hearing, sight and muscles of the face. An ophthalmological consult is seriously recommended for treatment to the eye on the side of the shingles to prevent blindness. Valtrex is the treatment of choice and is given 500mg three times a day for one week.

Prevention of Shingles

It is strongly recommended to get a recombinant zoster vaccine (RZV) vaccine (also known as Shingrix) after having shingles, and as a preventive vaccine starting at the age of 50. Postherpetic neuralgia is pain that occurs after the shingles outbreak and remains chronic. Sometimes the pain is severe and requires other medications such as Neurontin to keep the pain controlled.

RZV is a 2-dose series given 2-6 months apart. It is not a live vaccine, and has been recommended in October 2017 by the ACIP as the vaccine of choice to prevent Herpes Zoster, and given post-shingles for those 50 years and older, over Zostavax (live vaccine). It is kept frozen until administration, where it is diluted with a diluent and is given subcutaneously. The vaccine is expensive, and many doctor's offices do not carry it. You would need to get a prescription from your HCP and bring it to the pharmacy to dispense it.

Have the discussion with your HCP to make sure you are covered for this condition, as shingles does not come without complications for some: infection at the site, ulcers, and chronic pain that reduces the quality of life.

Laceration

A laceration is a cut or incision that involves multiple layers of tissue beneath the skin. Dermabond is a tissue adhesive that is applied in the emergency room to hold the skin together. If the laceration is very deep, absorbable stitches may need to be inserted in the lower tissues to keep the skin together. The important thing to do is to keep the area clean and dry, avoid soaking the area and avoid soap or ointments. If the laceration is not deep, steri-strips work well. This is the time to determine if a Tdap (tetanus shot with acellular pertussis) is needed. If it has been more than 10 years since the last Tdap vaccine, or you do not remember when it was last given, it is recommended to get one. Keep a record of this shot in your log book for the patient.

How to apply Steri-strips:

Steri-strips come on a card with a slit to help for easy removal.

- Cut them into halves if you wish
- To apply steri-strips to the skin, make sure the laceration is clean and dry.

- Apply one end of the steri-strip to the side of the laceration, about 1/4 inch from it. Pull the cut together so that the edges of the wound are touching each other.
- Then gently pull the steri-strip across and over the cut and adhere it to the other side of the laceration.
- Once the first steri-strip is secured, apply more until the laceration is completely covered.
- Apply a second layer and crisscross them for better adherence
- If the wound is in a moveable area such as the hand or the foot, apply a cut-up sock or a dressing to protect it
- Check under the dressing daily. If the wound has some drainage on it, change the dressing but leave the steri-strips intact
- Steri strips start to curl, get dry and fall off in a week
- To remove them, start on the top layer and gently peel them off before removing the bottom layer
- If steri strips are applied well, a laceration can heal without much of a scar

(Go to YouTube at Caregiver Success for the video on "Skin Tears")

Staples or Sutures

Head lacerations usually require staples to be inserted, in order for the skin on the head to completely heal. Sutures or sewing the laceration together may be needed, especially in a moveable area so that the wound does not come open. Depending on which was done, the staples or sutures could be removed by a home care nurse or your HCP in 7 to 10 days.

Sleep Problems (Insomnia)

As we get older, a good night's sleep can be hard to come by. If the person is not very active and snoozes in the chair throughout the day, it is hard to sleep all night. Aunt Annette said she would sleep four hours then get up at 2 AM, play solitaire for 3 hours, then go back to sleep till 11AM.

There are many reasons for insomnia: anxiety, depression, stress, and certain medications can be culprits for sleep deprivation. Antidepressants, steroids, pain relievers that contain caffeine (Midlothian, Excedrin), water pills, cold and flu medications are a few medications that can interfere with sleep. Medical problems such as asthma, acid reflux, chronic pain, and Parkinson's disease can also be contributing factors to reduce sleep.

It is important to look at daily habits such as drinking coffee late at night, or watching TV while in bed. Having the room dark, cool, some white noise like a fan, is an environment that can help with improving sleep. Eat your evening meal early, and avoid heavy foods two hours before bedtime. The American Academy of Sleep Medicine recommends that we stop drinking caffeinated drinks at least 6 hours before sleep.

There are a few supplements that are considered "natural" but can still have side effects and interfere with other medications, so check with your pharmacist before starting them. They are considered dietary supplements and the FDA does not regulate such substances.

Melatonin is a hormone that our bodies produce at night and is triggered when the sun goes down. It is not as effective in treating insomnia but can work for jet lag. Stay on the lower doses: 1 to 3 mg to reduce the chance of side effects and drowsiness the next day. It can be purchased over-the-counter.

Valerian is an herb used for centuries to treat anxiety and insomnia that has mild sedative effects, and they have different formulations. Valerian is considered to be safe and not habit forming. It works best if taken daily for 2 weeks. It can interfere with statins and antihistamines.

Chamomile is most effective for sleep when you bring water to a boil, add 2-3 tea bags to the water, cover with a lid and brew for 10 minutes.

Tryptophan is actually an amino acid used to form serotonin, which is a substance in the brain that tells your body to fall asleep. Its byproduct is L-tryptophan, which can help you fall asleep faster.

Lavender used in a diffuser has a soothing effect when inhaled. I have used it in the evening for calming reasons.

Over-the-counter sleep aids have antihistamines as their primary ingredient that help with sleep. Nytol, Sominex have diphenhydramine; and Unisom, Nighttime Sleep Aid contains doxylamine. Other OTC sleep aids such as Tylenol PM and NyQuil contain Tylenol and alcohol respectively. Side effects of these drugs are:

- Drowsiness the next day
- Forgetfulness
- Feeling off balance with the chance of falling
- Dry mouth
- Constipation and urinary retention

Sleeping pills that are newer, that have fewer side effects, with less dependency and are still controlled substances include Sonata, Ambien (Zolpidem), and Lunesta.

Their side effects include:

- Drug tolerance
- Rebound insomnia

SLEEP PROBLEMS (INSOMNIA)

- Headache, dizziness, nausea, difficulty swallowing
- Worsening depression with suicidal thoughts

The Mayo Clinic has free E-newsletters you can subscribe to and receive bi-weekly readings about various up-to-date medical topics, such as insomnia.

HelpGuide.org Insomnia *What to Do When You Can't Sleep,* L. Robinson, M. Smith M.A., R. Segal, M.A. 9/2018).

Here are some other helpful ideas to improve on sleep: eat a light eat meal of mostly carbohydrates or tryptophan 2-3 hours before sleep: have pasta, lentils, potatoes, or cereal. Do not look at screens, such as TV or iPhones but read a book or stare at the ceiling to get "into the zone." Keeping a positive attitude, like "I will sleep tonight," not "another night of not sleeping," will help sleep.

There is a device called "Dodow." It is a small circular object, that is placed on your nightstand. When touched, it emits a light blue light on the ceiling. By focusing on this exterior signal, it draws attention away from other distractions that are floating through your psyche. By doing so, your respiratory rate is reduced from 11-6 breaths per minute, and ideal sleep is reached in 8 minutes. If you should wake up during the night, just touch the screen again and repeat the process.

Sprains and Strains

A sprain is a painful injury to a joint or joints due to a partial or complete tear of ligaments.

What should you do?
Here is a great mnemonic: **R-I-C-E**: **R**ice **I**ce **C**ompression **E**levation

- For the first 24 hours, keep the injured limb raised on 2 pillows while lying down. Apply a bag of frozen peas or ice wrapped in a towel to the limb every 2 hours for 20 to 30 minutes. Do this only while awake because you should not leave ice on a limb unattended to prevent frostbite.
- Take Tylenol every 4 hours or Advil (with food) every 6 hours for pain or discomfort.
- An ACE bandage can be applied and removed every 3 to 4 hours. Apply the ACE firm enough but not too tight, to keep the swelling down. The best way to tell that the ACE is not too tight, watch the toes or fingers for swelling, bluish discoloration, coldness, numbness, or excessive pain. If you see these signs happen, loosen the ACE and reapply it immediately. Another trick is to be able to insert two fingers under the ACE, then you know it is not too tight.

(Look under Section 2: How to apply an Ace Wrap).

If there is persistent pain and the person is unable to use the injured area for more than 2 to 3 days, this may be a sign of a broken bone. A hairline fracture may not appear on an x-ray, but with a repeat x-ray a week later, or having the radiologist take another look at the original x-ray since there is no change in the person, the fracture may be seen.

Strains

A strain is when the muscles and ligaments are stretched. A strain can occur anywhere in the body. A neck injury, or cervical strain, is actually a "pain in the neck." An x-ray should be done to assure there is no fracture. If there is any weakness in moving arms or legs immediately after the injury, it is important to tell your HCP. The treatment to do is to apply ice such as a frozen gel pack or a bag of frozen peas wrapped in a towel, around the neck every 1-2 hours for 20 to 30 minutes at a time. A cervical collar can help support the neck as the strain heals. It is removed when showering or icing. Tylenol or Motrin can be given to help with pain relief.

X-rays are usually repeated in one week to ten days to make sure a hairline fracture is not overlooked. It is important that the person reports to your HCP if he:

- Has pain that is increasing in the neck
- Has difficulty swallowing or breathing
- Has difficulty walking
- Has developed numbness, weakness, or movement problems in the arms or legs
- Has developed problems with walking
- Has developed bowel or bladder retention or incontinence

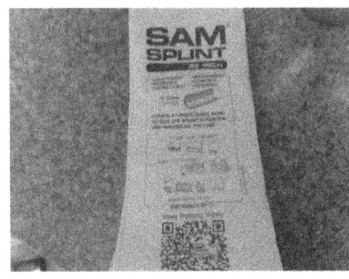

Compact splint device for immobilizing bone and soft tissue injuries

Stomach Problems

Bloating and Gas- what can you do to feel better?

The gut is called "our second brain." Stress and feelings such as "butterflies in the stomach" are caused by a nerve called the vagus nerve. Diarrhea versus constipation with bloating and feeling like you are going to "blow up" is common for many people. Some people complain of persistent reflux or belching causing them to be afraid to go out with friends for meals. They may also complain of frequent bathroom visits. Irritable bowel syndrome has become the common diagnosis, but it is good to have a full GI work up to rule out diverticulitis or Small Intestine Bacterial Overgrowth (SIBO).

Fermentable **O**ligosaccharides **D**isaccharides **M**onosaccharides **P**olyols, called **"FODMAPS"** is found in many foods we eat every day. It is the sugars that feed on the bad bacteria in your gut that can cause all of those digestive problems above. Many of this information is online, but here is a brief list of foods you can eat and foods you should avoid. You should try this food exercise for at least one week and see how you feel. Some people find it easy to follow, but there are some restrictions on what foods you should avoid.

Foods you CAN eat:

Bell peppers	Spinach
Carrots	Kale
Green beans	Tomato
Bok Choy	Zucchini
Cucumbers	Yams
Lettuce	Eggplant

Olives- green and black
Ginger
Potatoes- sweet and regular
Mozzarella cheese
Parmesan cheese
Swiss and cheddar cheese
Butternut Squash
Rice- brown and white
Oats
Quinoa
Gluten-free bread and pasta
Almond milk

Fruit juice- not from concentrate
All meats/fish
Almonds
Peanuts
Oranges
Honeydew
Cantaloupe
Blueberries
Grapefruit
Kiwi
Lemon
Strawberries

Foods you should AVOID:

Garlic
Cabbage
Broccoli
Cauliflower
Snow peas
Asparagus
Sweet corn
Brussel sprouts
Mushrooms of all kinds
Peaches

Nectarines
Plums
Apples
Watermelon
Peas
Blackberries
Pistachios
Ice cream
Raisins
Avocado (small amounts)

Leaky Gut- what is that??

Leaky Gut Syndrome is where the one cell lining of the intestines becomes penetrable, allowing toxic bacteria and partially digested food proteins into the bloodstream. These are considered to be foreign invaders, and the body detects them, triggering the immune system.

Nine Signs of Leaky Gut:

1. Digestive issues such as gas, bloating, diarrhea or irritable bowel syndrome
2. Food allergies or food intolerances
3. Brain fog, difficulty concentrating, ADHD
4. Mood imbalances such as depression and anxiety
5. Skin issues such as acne, rosacea or eczema
6. Seasonal allergies or asthma
7. Hormonal imbalances such as irregular periods, PMS (pre-menstrual syndrome), or polycystic ovarian syndrome (PCOS)
8. Diagnosis of an autoimmune disease such as rheumatoid arthritis, Hashimoto's thyroiditis, lupus, psoriasis, or celiac disease
9. Diagnosis of chronic fatigue or fibromyalgia

What causes Leaky Gut?

- This syndrome can develop for several reasons:
- Antibiotic use, corticosteroids, radiation, alcohol consumption, smoking, obesity, chemotherapy, and the contraceptive pill.
- Food (gluten, dairy, and other toxic and inflammatory foods (see foods to avoid above under Fodmap diet)
- Gut infections (candida overgrowth, (small intestinal bacterial overgrowth (SIBO)
- Toxins (medications, mercury, pesticides)
- Stress (chronic emotional or physical stress)

Some things you can do to improve gut health:

- Follow the Fodmap diet
- Avoid the bad habits above, e.g., smoking, etc.
- Reduce stress - consider yoga, meditation, exercise
- Take pre- and probiotics

Heartburn- understanding how to treat it

What does it feel like? Usually, people complain that they have a burning sensation in the middle of the chest. It usually occurs after eating. Sometimes the person has a bitter or after-taste with increased chest burning when lying down. It is caused by the lower esophageal sphincter (LES) to relax and allow the stomach acid to enter the esophagus.

Heartburn (also known as GERD - Gastric Esophageal Reflux Disease) when more serious, can be caused by a number of foods and beverages:

- Alcohol
- Coffee
- Fried or fatty foods
- Spicy or acidic foods
- Onions
- Chocolate
- Mint
- Caffeine
- Smoking

Some other causes of GERD are:
- Obesity where the stomach is pressing up on the diaphragm causing the LES to open and allowing acid to go into the esophagus. Losing weight could be the best solution for many people!
- Hiatal hernia- a protrusion of part of the stomach through the diaphragm. If the hernia is small, the symptoms will probably be mild; but if it is large, there are bigger symptoms.

The problems you can experience are:

- Regurgitation of food in the mouth
- Acid reflux
- Difficulty swallowing
- Chest or abdominal pain
- Shortness of breath
- Vomiting of blood or passing of black stools, which may mean gastrointestinal bleeding so **call 911**!

How to treat heart burn

Everyone can experience this problem occasionally, but it is when it becomes consistent that medication may be needed. By removing foods that irritate your gut and considering over-the-counter H2 blockers like Prilosec or Protonix, you can eliminate the symptoms.

What else can you do to avoid symptoms?

- Avoid lying down for 3 hours after eating
- Stop smoking
- Keep the head of the bed elevated 4-6 inches to prevent acid from moving up into the esophagus

- Lose excess weight (reducing the belly size, can reduce the pressure on the LES)
- Sleep on your left side
- Eat smaller meals
- Limit carbonated beverages and gassy foods like broccoli and cabbage
- Avoid foods on the list above

If the symptoms persist, it would be good to see a gastroenterologist to look down into the esophagus and stomach to check for inflammation or stomach ulcers. If there is a hiatal hernia, then surgery may be necessary to tighten the LES.

Is it a heart burn or a heart attack?

- Heart burn is a burning pain in the stomach or chest soon after eating
- The pain usually does not radiate to the neck, shoulders, or arms
- Pain is quickly relieved when taking an antacid (like TUMS)

Is it a heart attack or angina?

- A dull or crushing pressure in the center of the chest, usually a tight feeling
- Often occurs with activity or exertion
- Pain can spread to the neck, shoulders, and arms
- Usually, a person is sweating and feels like it is hard to breathe
- Can have nausea and vomiting.
- If the person has these symptoms, give an aspirin 325mg to chew and **call 911**!

(Adapted from ACIP 2004)

Nausea and Vomiting

The question is:

- how long have you had these symptoms?
- do you have a fever?
- does anyone you live with or have recently seen have the same symptoms?

If so, it is most likely viral and will resolve on its own in 48 hours.

The person you would worry the most about is the person who is frail and has little reserve. This person becomes dehydrated quickly and would need IV hydration; hence hospitalization.

The best thing to do is to:

- stay home in bed
- drink clear fluids including tea
- avoid dairy products
- avoid vegetables
- eat bland foods like toast with jelly in small amounts
- take Pepto Bismol to soothe the stomach
- take Tylenol for fever
- be patient and let the condition run its course

For an older person, give chicken broth, Gatorade or Jell-O. Encourage small, frequent sips of fluids. Observe that the person is urinating as this will tell you that they are getting hydrated.

Signs of dehydration:

- Dry eyes that look sunken
- Urine is small amounts and dark in color
- Feeling thirstier than usual

- A new fever occurs
- Vomiting blood or coffee grounds

Appendicitis

The appendix is a small pouch of the colon that projects on the right side of the abdomen. The appendix becomes infected by bacteria, becomes inflamed then fills with pus.

Appendicitis can mimic a stomach bug in the beginning. The person complains of nausea and vomiting, low-grade fever, abdominal bloating and loss of appetite. The only difference is there is sudden pain around the navel that then moves down the right side of the abdomen. Also, no one else is sick like you in the house. The usual age is between 20 and 30, but it can occur in older people. The standard treatment is surgical removal.

For an older person and for someone who becomes suddenly ill, this condition warrants a **911** call. My brother-in-law developed a ruptured appendix and needed to be hospitalized for 10 days for complications after surgery. If there is a suspicion it may be appendicitis, call 911 or see your HCP immediately.

Diverticulitis

A diverticulum is a small pouch or sac located on the colon. During a colonoscopy, the large intestine is visualized, and these pouches can be seen. Sometimes there are a few, and sometimes, there are many. Diverticulosis is the name of this condition, but diverticulitis occurs when the pouch gets filled with bacteria, as well as food. This situation causes pressure in the diverticulum and leads to infection and inflammation.

The symptoms include left-sided abdominal pain. The person can experience fever, bloating, nausea, vomiting, and diarrhea. It was thought that seeds and nuts can aggravate this condition but that turned out to be a false claim. You may need blood work to check your white count for elevation, a CAT scan of the abdomen and urine check to make sure the abdominal pain is not from some other condition.

Treatment

The person may need:

- Intravenous fluids
- Pain and nausea medications
- To rest the bowels by having only liquids for a few days followed by soft, easily digestible foods

To prevent recurrence of diverticulitis:

- Maintain a high fiber diet
- Chose bran-based cereals or oatmeal
- Add wheat germ to dishes
- Eat whole grain bread over white bread
- Eat fruit instead of drinking fruit juice- as you get the skin and the pulp= more fiber!
- Enjoy healthy snacks: popcorn, whole grain crackers, nuts, and carrot sticks

Seek immediate medical attention if:

- Pain does not improve or worsens
- Bowel movements do not return to normal
- Oral temperature goes above 102, even with Tylenol
- Black or bloody stools with tarry consistency

If the diverticulum ruptures, the person will need emergency surgery- **call 911!**

Hernia- what is it?

There is more than one type of hernia. We discussed the hiatal hernia above.

The umbilical hernia is located at the navel, and is a result of part of the bowel looping out, causing an "outie belly button." It usually happens after birth, but can develop later on due to obesity, previous abdominal surgery, and multiple pregnancies. This hernia can stay quiet and can occur in middle-aged obese men who present with acute pain at the navel with a ring of redness around it. This warrants immediate surgery for most, as the bowel is now incarcerated, or strangulated, preventing the passage of stool and leading to a bowel blockage.

Inguinal Hernia

An inguinal hernia is a bulge noted in the groin caused by a small part of the intestine protruding through a weak spot in the abdominal muscles. It can remain intact without causing pain, for years. In a male, the bulge may move down into the scrotum. If it can be pushed back into the groin, it is called "reduceable," and is not of concern. If it becomes painful, fever develops, nausea or vomiting occurs, or inability to have a bowel movement occurs, the hernia could be strangulated warranting a **911 call.**

Stroke- What is it and what are the symptoms

One of my patients was only 48 years old when he had a massive stroke leaving his right side paralyzed. He had a history of hypertension and diabetes but did go for medical check-ups. Both he and his wife were teachers, did not have children. They were looking forward to retirement in the next 5 years. They traveled, and built their home together while working full-time. They were inseparable. Their lives were changed forever.

Bob was in rehabilitation to learn to walk and talk again. He was fitted with expensive equipment, such as a tilt-in-space wheelchair, and other necessary equipment so he could be cared for at home. Deb gave up her job to care for Bob, and took early retirement. She was his 24/7 companion for over 25 years when he died at home at the age of 73 years old.

As his clinician for over 6 years and saw how hard it was on Deb. Due to the stroke, Bob could not speak clearly and had limited use of the left side. We worked together bringing in the community to help her. It was not an easy experience for any of us. What I am trying to say is, it is important to get regular medical care, and know not to wait to assess if what you are experiencing was truly a stroke; because the window of opportunity to reverse the symptoms is limited.

There actually two types of strokes: hemorrhagic and ischemic. Both are a medical emergency and require a 911 call. Hemorrhagic strokes are less common, only causing about 15% of strokes, but are responsible for 40% of deaths. Either an aneurysm bursts or there is a leak in a small blood vessel in the brain. The blood spills into the tissues causing swelling and pressure.

This is called an intracerebral hemorrhage. Some of the brain cells become damaged and die, affecting the proper function of part of the brain. The other type of brain bleed is called a subarachnoid hemorrhage. The bleeding occurs between the brain and the tissue covering it, called the subarachnoid space. Blood thinners, head injury or a bleeding disorder, can cause this type of hemorrhage.

An ischemic stroke is when a blood vessel in the brain is blocked by a blood clot. The cause of this type of stroke is from hypertension. There are two types of ischemic strokes: embolic and thrombotic. An embolic stroke is caused by atrial fibrillation and occurs in 15 % of people. A plaque or blood clot travels to the brain and blocks a small blood vessel. This blood clot is called an embolus. The second type of stroke is caused by a blood clot that forms inside an artery in the brain. People with high cholesterol tend to get this type of stroke. This type of clot is called a thrombus.

Some symptoms of a stroke are:

- Sudden numbness or weakness of the face, arm or leg- especially one side of the body
- Sudden droopiness of the face on one side- you cannot smile or raise one eyebrow on one side
- Sudden change in vision: you see double in one or both eyes, blurriness or you see a blackened area
- Sudden headache with or without vomiting and dizziness
- Sudden loss of balance or coordination
- Sudden trouble speaking, or understanding speech

Note the time the symptoms started, and tell the paramedics this information. Going to a stroke center in your community is necessary to look for a bleed in the brain or a clot so they can decide how to treat it right away. A stroke can be reversible but needs to be addressed immediately. If the stroke is not treated quickly, the physical disability can be permanent.

What is a TIA?

A TIA (transient ischemic attack) also known as a "mini-stroke" is a stroke that lasts for only a few minutes. It happens when the blood supply to the brain is temporarily stopped due to a blood clot.

There are actually 3 reasons that can cause TIA:

1. Low blood flow at a narrow part of a major artery carrying blood to the brain such as in a carotid artery
2. A blood clot breaks off from somewhere else in the body and travels to the brain, blocking off a blood vessel
3. The third is a narrowing of a smaller blood vessel in the brain usually caused by build-up of plaque (a fatty substance).

The symptoms are the same as those listed above for a stroke but do not last as long and with full recovery within the next 24 hours. A mini-stroke is a warning sign that a bigger, more permanent stroke may occur in the future. The time table could be the next few hours, days or months.

Syncope (Fainting Episode)

A fainting episode is a sudden, short-lived loss of consciousness. It results in you having a complete recovery and is attributed to a temporary shortage of oxygen and/or glucose to the brain.

What are the causes of syncope?

- Blood pressure pills or other medications that can lower your blood pressure below normal
- Sudden changes in posture, like standing up too fast
- Standing too long, where blood pools in the legs and feet
- Seizure disorder
- Fear of the sight of blood
- Irregular heartbeat
- Hardening of the arteries where the brain temporarily does not receive enough blood
- Bearing down when going to the bathroom. Your blood pressure will suddenly rise, and your body compensates by making your blood pressure drop too low when you stop bearing down (Valsalva Maneuver)
- Low blood sugar

Seek IMMEDIATE Medical Attention by calling **911** if:

- If you have another fainting spell
- If you have chest pain, nausea or vomiting
- You have a loss of feeling in some part of your body or lose movement in your arms or legs

- You have difficulty talking
- You become sweaty or feel light headed

A syncopal episode can be very scary to observe. My husband, Steve, had one after having a total hip replacement and tried to get up too fast while in the bathroom. He actually fell backwards landing in the shower stall. Luckily, the new hip was not compromised and he did not fracture any bones.

His eyes were wide open staring at me, not blinking, and he was not responding for about 45 seconds. I immediately checked his pulse, which was weak, and started calling his name. I applied a wet towel on his head and slapped his face. I called for his daughter, and when he became conscious, he said everything just went black.

Post-surgery and anesthesia, especially something as invasive as a hip replacement, warrants care when trying to sit up. Our mistake was not going home with the urinal. It would have allowed Steve to stay in bed the first 24 hours and use the urinal without getting up. I can only imagine the complications he could have had: needing surgery again, fractured limbs or back, or neck…. The list could go on.

(View my YouTube channel, "Caregiver Success" to watch a series of videos on having a Mako Total Hip Replacement")

Thyroid Disease

The thyroid gland, like other organs in our body as we age, begins to work less efficiently. The thyroid is a gland shaped like a butterfly and sits right below your Adam's apple on either side of your windpipe (throat area). It has been called "our body clock." The purpose of the thyroid is to make and store thyroid hormone into your blood, which affects every cell in our body. When the thyroid is sluggish, you feel tired; your skin is dry, heartbeat slows, you could become depressed, constipated and sleepy. This condition is called hypothyroidism.

On the other hand, when your thyroid is overactive, the opposite happens: the heart is racing, you are nervous, lose weight, have diarrhea and can't sleep. This condition is called hyperthyroidism. When the person has multiple symptoms, as mentioned above, a TSH (Thyroid Stimulating Hormone) blood test will help determine if the thyroid is malfunctioning.

TSH is released from the pituitary gland (in the brain) and regulated by the hypothalamus (also in the brain) when the thyroid hormone is low. When it is released, it causes your thyroid to make more thyroid hormone. So, with hypothyroidism, the blood test will show an elevated TSH, and the opposite when you have hyperthyroidism. It is a little confusing but makes sense when you think about it.

Synthroid (or levothyroxine) is the medication prescribed and adjusted so that the thyroid works better. Armour thyroid medication contains T3 and T4 hormones obtained from pig thyroid. Thyroid medications are to be taken first thing in the morning, 30 minutes before a meal or other medications. The medication is taken for life. Once you have the diagnosis of hypothyroidism, it is good to have a TSH checked regularly to make sure the medication is working well. Getting too much Synthroid is as bad as getting too little.

Hyperthyroidism can also occur but is not as popular as hypothyroidism. If left untreated, serious problems with the bones (osteoporosis), and heart (irregular heart rate) leading to blood clots and stroke can occur. It is important to see your HCP to be diagnosed and you may need to see an endocrinologist who treats glandular disorders. Methimazole is an anti-thyroid agent used to treat hyperthyroidism.

Upper Respiratory Infection

It starts with a runny nose, headache and fatigue followed by night time cough. The common cold is caused by a virus so antibiotics will not cure it. The common cold, in an older person who is frail and has lung problems or a poor immune system, can quickly develop bronchitis or pneumonia. The mucus starts out clear, turns whiter, and after a week of symptoms, the phlegm can turn green. If the symptoms are improving, then this green phlegm just means we were approaching the end of a viral infection.

How to treat it:

Encourage fluids. This can be Jell-O, ice cream, chicken broth… water is not all that interesting in the older person due to a change in taste buds. In fact, most older people prefer sweet foods. Did you know that the tip of the tongue, when you lick a lollipop or ice cream cone, is where the sweet taste bud is?

Start a mucolytic such as Robitussin, Mucinex 12-hour or liquid Mucinex. Use as directed on the bottle. Remember to look for sugarless versions if the person is diabetic. Another remedy which is homeopathic is Cold-EEZE lozenges. Sucking on six a day reduces the effects of the rhinovirus, therefore, reduces cold symptoms. Only use lozenges if the person does not have a history of choking or swallowing issues!

Nasal saline and the use of a humidifier can increase the moisture in the nasal passages to help whisk away germs as well as loosen secretions. It is important to clean the humidifier regularly so it does not become a reservoir of germs. The same is true for a neti-pot which is used to flush out the sinuses. Always use distilled water, not tap water because the tap water has bacteria in it.

Laryngitis

If the person had a recent cold and now cannot speak, she may have laryngitis. She first may have had a post nasal drip which could cause the vocal cords to be inflamed. Start a mucolytic such as Tussin or Robitussin. Avoid ones with sugar and Sudafed if the person has diabetes or high blood pressure, respectively. Gargles with 8 oz of warm water with 1 teaspoon of salt 4x/day, as well as avoiding talking or whispering until her voice comes back. Keep the sleeve warm at all times. It has been postulated that the warm moist heat draws out the virus from the throat. Cold-EEZE is throat lozenges that work great if Mom can suck on 6/day. Soups, ice cream, apple sauce, and any soft foods are encouraged while swallowing is painful. Liquids will help loosen up the secretions so they can be coughed up.

Sinusitis

A virus can settle anywhere in our respiratory tract; either in the throat, lungs or sinuses. When a person says it hurts around the eyes or she has a frontal headache, assume there may be a sinus infection. Pressing on the cheeks or forehead to elicit pain will help to locate the inflammation. We also have very small sinuses called ethmoid sinuses near the nasal areas of both eyes. These sinuses do not drain well and can cause eye pain. The person may also be dizzy and feel like she is "in a cloud." Treatment for a sinus infection depends on how long she has had it, what color is the phlegm, and how much phlegm she has.

Always start with some type of mucolytic. If the older person can take Mucinex (guaifenesin), which is a 12-hour pill (and easier for compliance) have her start taking it. Avoid getting Mucinex that has sudafed or alcohol. Drink plenty of clear fluids during the day. Warm soup is great. Try to avoid antibiotics as they do not treat a virus and will affect the gut flora.

Warm moist compresses will help soothe the sinuses. If the person has a fever of 100.4 oral or higher and green phlegm early in the symptoms, she may have a bacterial infection. Now, consider antibiotics. If the phlegm turns green on day 8 of being sick, it is usually the remains of an old viral infection, which could last up to 14 days.

If a nasal spray is in order such as Nasonex, Dymysta or Flonase, for example, there is a right way and wrong way to take it. When I teach people how to use a nasal spray - I use a rhyme. "Blow your nose and look at your toes."

Picture the sinuses- the maxillary sinuses are small pockets on either side of the nose. When your head is leaning forward, and you clear your nose by blowing first, the medication has a place to be absorbed. After all, we breathe in, and all the allergens come in through the nose.

Then with the head tilted forward, cover the right nostril with the left hand, squirt one or two sprays in the left nostril, then reverse the process. Keep your head forward as you immediately snuff the medication in through the nose. Do not put your head back, because "if you tasted it, you wasted it." This means the medication went down the throat and is no longer in the sinuses.

A Neti-pot or Sinu cleanse are great nasal cleansers. It looks like a genie bottle with a tiny spout at the end. You can buy them in any pharmacy or grocery store. You can buy salt packets or make saltwater yourself.

How to use Sinucleanse:

- Fill the pot to the line with warm **distilled** water.
- Add the salt packet to the water and gently stir the bottle.
- Over a sink with your head forward, turn head, left cheek down
- Insert the spout into the right nostril
- You will feel warm water moving over the nasal bridge and come out the other nostril
- Blow your nose if you wish
- Switch nostrils
- When you have a cold or suffer from allergies, wash out of the sinuses once a day. It will remove germs and allergens.

Urinary Tract Conditions

Urinary Incontinence

There are many types of urinary incontinence. Through various blood work, studies, and patient's symptoms a urologist can determine the cause.

Let's go through them:

Transient Reversible Incontinence

This condition is when the person who was able to control her urine is now having episodes of incontinence. It may be caused by a urinary tract infection, and when treated the incontinence is reversed.

Functional Incontinence

This form of incontinence is when a person is aware of the need to urinate, but for a physical or mental reason, they are unable to get to void. There could be a small amount of urinary leakage with the inability to fully empty the bladder.

How do we help this type of incontinence?

- Order physical or occupational therapy
- Evaluate environmental barriers such as clutter on the way to the bathroom
- Habit training- regularly prompted voiding
- Wear absorbent pads or briefs

Stress or Urge Incontinence

This type of incontinence is mostly found in women in which urine is released after a cough or jumping. Kegel exercises involve repeatedly contracting the pelvic floor muscles. If done repeatedly and frequently for 3 months, it can reduce the symptoms of stress incontinence. Medications to treat this condition are Myrbetriq, Ditropan, Toviaz, Vesicare, Flonase, and Terazosin to name a few.

Overflow Incontinence

This form of incontinence is caused by an overfull bladder causing leaking of urine without the urge to urinate. An enlarged prostate gland, causes a blockage of the bladder outlet, or the muscle that allows urine to be released is too weak to a to empty the bladder normally.

How to improve this condition:

- Use a urinary catheter and intermittently remove the urine
- Surgery may be necessary to remove the obstruction
- Medications such as Urecholine and Proscar work if there is no obstruction

Mixed/ Stress/ Urge Incontinence

Mostly a problem for the older woman. Treat the worst symptom first.

Urinary Tract Infection (UTI)

UTI is a medical problem that is very common in the older person, especially in women. The fact that the woman's urethra, which is the tube where the urine comes out, is short, the chance of organisms invading this tube is great. One bad habit some women have is wiping from the back near the rectum to the front. By doing so, the rectal flora is brought forward causing urethral contamination. The common organism found in a UTI is E Coli. This organism is predominantly found in the rectum.

When a woman wears an undergarment due to incontinence, the wet garment if left on too long can lead to a UTI. A UTI is an infection that occurs anywhere between the kidneys and the urethra, and most of the time involves the bladder. Also, soaking in the tub can lead to a bladder infection. Having a Foley catheter increases the risk for a UTI since the body sees it as a foreign body.

For a man, an enlarged prostate gland can cause infection as well. The prostate gland is like a donut with a hole in it. It wraps around the urethra and sits below the bladder. If it is large, it can squeeze the urethra, causing urine to back up into the bladder leading to a UTI. A man would say he cannot urinate or that he has to push to get any urine out. There are medications that can help make the prostate smaller. A Prostate Specific Antigen (PSA) blood test would indicate whether there are some issues with the prostate, as well as palpating the prostate gland through the rectum.

A CAT scan of the kidneys could reveal stones. Stones are caused by crystal-forming substances such as calcium oxalate and uric acid. When a person does not drink enough fluids, the crystals collect and begin forming stones. They can be present in the kidney, ureter (the tube that leads from the kidney to the bladder), or in the bladder. They can cause severe pain in the back and can radiate to the lower abdomen and groin. They are also a reason UTIs occur. A stent may be placed, which is a small tube to relieve swelling and promote healing. (Mayo Clinic 2018)

There is a urinalysis test that can be ordered with a reflex test. The reflex test can show different results:

- Leukocyte esterase alone
- White blood cells over 5 high power field (HPF) alone
- Presence of yeast
- Presence of bacteria AND presence of white blood cells greater than 5 HPF
- OR leukocyte esterase, nitrites AND white blood cells greater than 5 HPF

Urine test strips you can purchase at a pharmacy to test urine at home for a UTI. These strips are for UTI testing only and will tell you there is an infection, but a urine culture would still need to go to the lab to determine what organism exists.

Bacterial Colonization of Urine

Sometimes the level of bacteria in the urine will be high but there will be no physical symptoms. It is crucial not to treat with an antibiotic so quickly. After having multiple UTIs, the urine will colonize. They only time the urine should be treated is if there are symptoms. There are other preventive products and means to help reduce UTIs. They are mentioned further in this chapter.

Symptoms of UTI:

- the person's behavior changes- sleeping a lot, not eating, confused, falling
- urine has a foul odor

- you may see blood in the urine
- complaints of burning as the urine is coming down. If the pain is at the end of voiding, the bladder is infected; if the pain is during urination, then the urethra is infected.

Treatment:

A urine specimen is needed to look for blood and nitrites. A urine culture and sensitivity are crucial so that you can find out what the bacterial colony count is. If it is over 100,000, then this is a true UTI. The culture would tell you what the organism is, which is usually is E. Coli, but there could be more than one organism present. The sensitivity tells you which drug will fight the bug. Without a culture, you really do not know which antibiotic will take care of it.

Once the antibiotic is prescribed, it is important to complete it. It is also a good idea to start a probiotic, because the good flora in the gut is reduced for almost 9 months after taking an antibiotic. Sometimes Pyridium is ordered if the bladder infection is painful, as this medication is a pain reliever. Pyridium will turn the urine orange, so do not get alarmed. Obtaining a repeat urine specimen to check if the UTI is cleared is not always prudent. If the person is looking and feeling better after completion of the antibiotic, repeating the urine culture will not give you useful information.

Treating a UTI with antibiotics is not always the answer. The bug (organism) gets smarter each time an antibiotic is given. It becomes more resistant to antibiotics, as it mutates. Eventually, with long-term use of oral antibiotics, many can only be given by intravenous and can lead to antibiotic resistance. Try to abstain from antibiotics as much as possible and use good, clean care with toileting.

URINARY TRACT INFECTION (UTI)

Urine Collection:

Here is how to collect a urine specimen for a continent male:

1. Wash your hands and apply gloves
2. Obtain a specimen cup
3. Take off the specimen lid and place it inner lid side up on the counter, avoid touching the inside of the lid
4. Use either a clean washcloth with liquid soap and water or a wet wipe
5. Clean the tip of the penis with a soapy washcloth then rinse the cloth with water and clean the penis again to remove soap, or use a new wet wipe. If there is a foreskin, push the foreskin back and clean the tip of the penis.
6. Do not touch the penis to the cup
7. Have the stream of urine start in the toilet then collect the middle of the stream (called midstream) into the cup
8. Put about 3 inches of urine into the cup
9. Replace the lid carefully without touching the inside of the lid10.Screw the lid on tight, put patient name on the cup, place it in a zip lock bag to
10. Make sure your HCP has sent a script over to the lab, or the lab will not take the specimen. It needs to get to the lab within 48 hours. A urine culture will take about 48 hours to get the final report.

It is not that easy to get a urine specimen from a person who is incontinent. For a man, there is such an item called a condom or male external catheter. It is connected to an extension tube and then to a leg bag. One company that makes the condom catheters is Freedom (Coloplast) 35 mm or 28mm (Ref 8400/8430) online. A latex-free extension tubing is made by Bard Ref #150615. The urinary leg bag 600 ccs by Dynarex (#4281). You will also need a urine specimen cup with a lid.

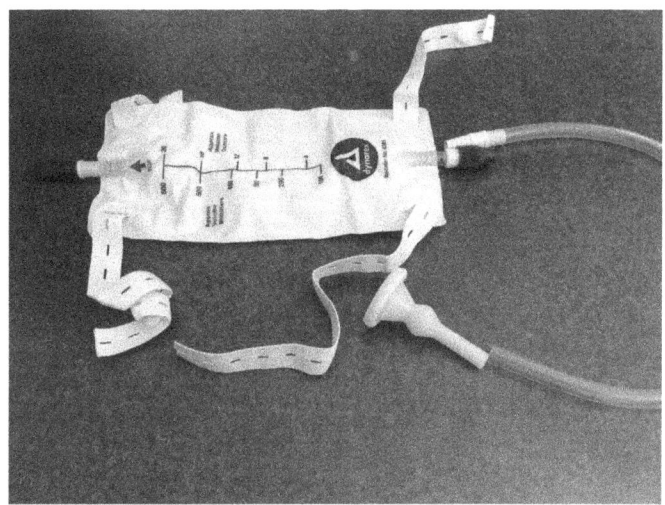

Here's how to collect a urine specimen for an incontinent male:

Follow steps 1 through 5 above then continue the steps below:

6. Put the condom catheter on the tip of the penis and gently roll it up the shaft of the penis
7. It is sticky so will adhere to the skin on the penis
8. Attach the extension tubing to the catheter being careful not to yank on the catheter
9. Attach the other end of the extension tubing to the leg bag.
10. Make sure to turn the spout on the end of the leg bag clockwise to tighten it to prevent urine from coming out.
11. Encourage fluids and collect a clean urine specimen
12. Open the lid from the urine cup and face it lid side up on the counter
13. Avoid touching the inside of the cup or lid with the collection leg bag
14. Turn the end of the spout counterclockwise for the urine to flow from the bag
15. Allow the urine to flow into the cup- up to 3 inches
16. Remove the condom catheter and discard it

URINARY TRACT INFECTION (UTI)

If a condom catheter is not anatomically going to work, consider using a SpeediCath Compact Set for males made by Coloplast. It is a sterile catheter that has a hydrophilic sheath and a collection bag. It is inserted into the penis to the bladder to collect a sterile urine specimen. The tip is Coude which means it is curved at the end so that it can be easily inserted. These catheters reduce the chance of getting a UTI over the traditional catheter. You can call Coloplast at 888-726-7872 and get a product catalog and some samples to try.

Here is how to collect a urine specimen from a continent female:

1. Wash your hands and apply gloves
2. Remove the specimen lid and place lid face up on the counter, avoid touching the inside
3. Use either a clean washcloth with liquid soap and water or 3 wet wipes
4. Clean the outer part of the vaginal area (left and right labia, and down the center of the vaginal area using a separate wipe for each area
5. Rinse the washcloth with water, or get new wet wipes to clean the outside and down the center
6. Start the stream of urine in the toilet, then collect the midstream of urine into the cup- about 3 inches
7. Replace the lid carefully on the cup
8. Screw the lid on tight, label name, DOB

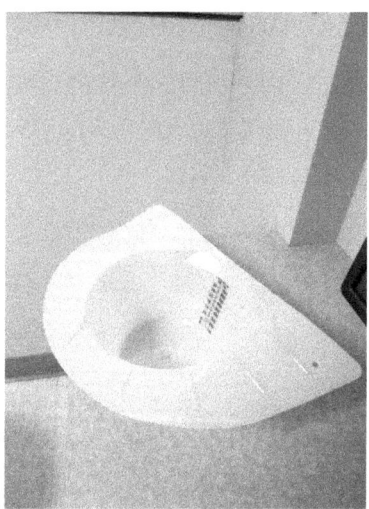

If the person is continent, you may want to use a "hat" to collect the urine. It is a plastic device that sits on the toilet under the rim. It is used once then is discarded. To get a good specimen, a female needs to spread the legs and aim the cup to collect the urine. This is not an easy task for an older woman to do without falling. It would make it easier to get a clean specimen, even midstream because the person can sit down, and the cup can be held between the legs.

Once the specimen is obtained, put the person's name on the specimen container, put it in a zip lock bag and place it in the refrigerator. Make sure your HCP has sent a script over to the lab, or the lab will not take the specimen. It needs to get to the lab within 48 hours. A urine culture will take about 48 hours to get the final report.

There is also a urine collection device for women I found in a camping store "for those on the go who just have to go" called "Lady J." I found it quite amusing because it is a plastic opening with a spout that is attached to a urinal which was advertised to be used for hot air balloonists, truckers, saleswomen, etc. The device is quite functional; therefore, it is another way of collecting urine. It can be purchased on Pilots HQ website under First Defense Industries at 888-798-4479.

How to collect a urine specimen from an incontinent female:

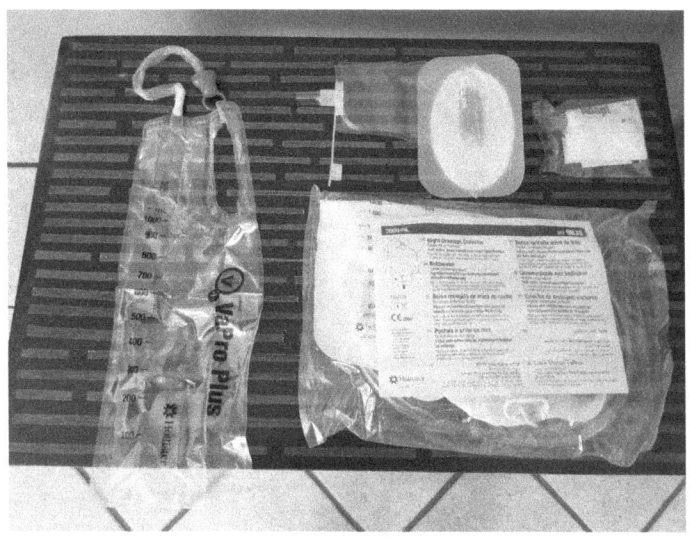

There is a urine collection device from Hollister that is used for bedridden patients. For a female or male who is bedridden, this product may be a good fit. You can call Hollister customer service M-F Central time at 1-888-808-7458 or request some samples of their products. Product #9811 is for the male urinary pouch and #9840 is for the female kit.

The pubic hair would need to be shaved off so the wafer can sit snugly on the skin. The beauty of this product is there is no catheter insertion, but a bag sits over the female perineum and over the penis of the male. It could be worn at night so that no none needs to get up at night for changing undergarments if it is not soiled from stool.

Another great product is called PureWick for females. This product is also good for day and night wear for the female who is not agitated because the device needs to stay in place. It is a "tampon" looking product that sits wedged between the legs where it absorbs urine. The urine is suctioned off the device into a cannister. It is made by Bard Medical through Liberator. The wicks last for 8-12 hour period. Call Bard Medical Customer service at 800-525-3467.

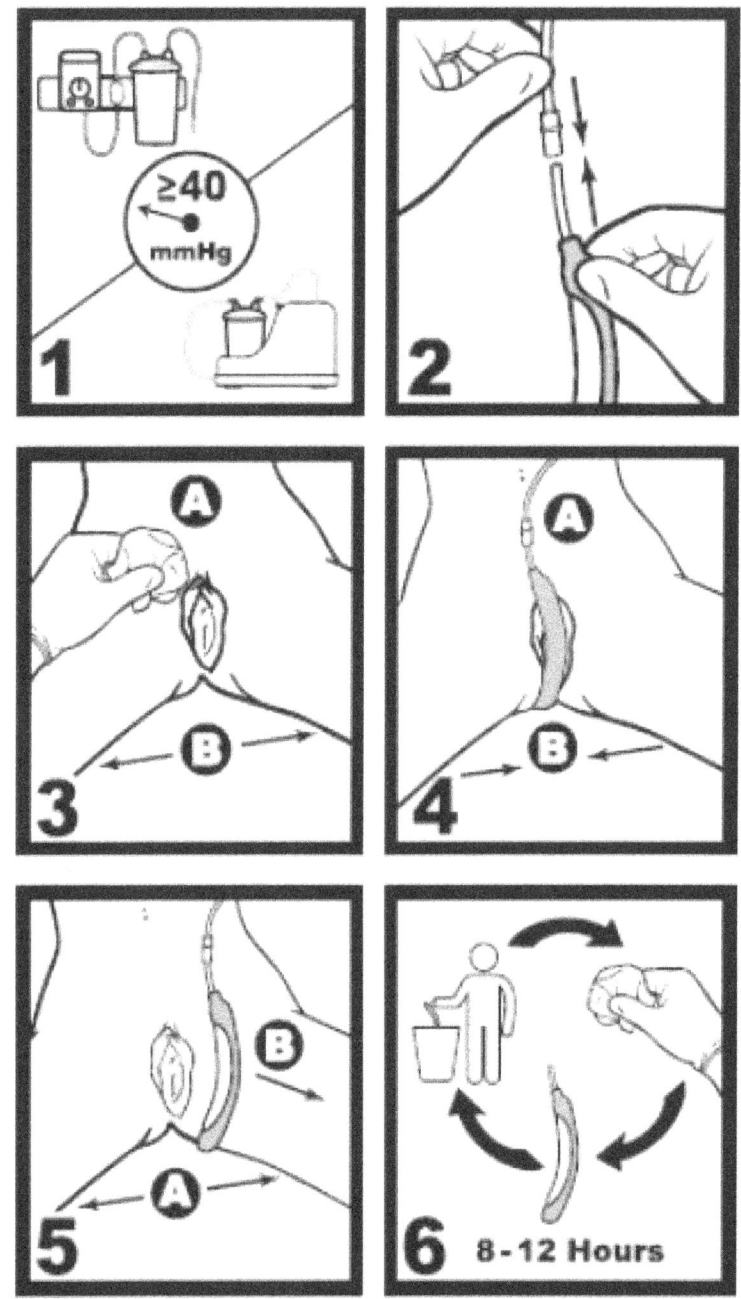

Application of a Purewick device

URINARY TRACT INFECTION (UTI)

Obtaining Urine from a Foley Catheter

Urine can be collected from a Foley catheter. This is called a "closed system," and the catheter and the bag should not be pulled apart to get urine. A visiting nurse could come to your home to help with this process or teach a reliable, teachable family member how to do it.

To obtain a specimen from this system, get:

- Specimen Cup
- Pair of gloves
- A syringe with needle
- Rubber band
- Alcohol wipe

Procedure:

- Have the person begin to take in more fluids so he can produce urine
- Clamp off the catheter just below the port on the catheter (the rubber raised circle on the foley)
- It may take an hour until there is enough urine to obtain
- Once you see urine in the tube above the port, you can try to get the specimen
- Open the specimen cup, and place the cap face up on the table
- Apply gloves
- Clean the port with an alcohol swab
- Insert the needle into the port and drawback to remove urine
- Place the urine into the specimen cup
- Repeat the last two steps until there are 2 inches of urine in the cup
- Once you have the urine, DO NOT FORGET TO REMOVE THE RUBBER BAND ON THE CATHETER so urine can flow
- Screw on the cap tightly and label the cup with person's name

What other types of catheters are there?

Coude Catheter

These catheters are used for self-catheterizing. A Coude catheter has a curved tip at the end. These catheters are prescribed for a man with an enlarged prostate gland. The curved tip makes it easier to insert the catheter past a tight area in the urethra. Women can also use them when they develop some blockage in the urethra. There are a variety of brands: Bard, Convatec, Coloplast, Hollister to name a few.

Intermittent Catheter

These are catheters to manage bladder drainage due to urinary retention, bladder obstruction or from neurological conditions that can cause paralysis or loss of sensation leading to incontinence. They are inserted and removed several times a day to drain urine. They replace the need for a continuous catheter and, so can reduce UTIs.

Straight Catheter

A straight catheter is used by individuals who have chronic bladder problems and can insert the catheter themselves. They can also be used to obtain a urine specimen.

Prevention of Urinary Tract Infection (UTI)

Many women that are now 80 and 90 years old were taught to wipe back to front. When doing this, fecal material is brought forward allowing the urethra to get exposed to it. It is hard for an older person to wipe the buttock from the back. She can be shown how to use a long-handled spoon of which a baby wipe can be wrapped around and secured using a rubber band. This way the person can reach the rectum and wipe separately from the front.

One other reason that UTIs and urinary incontinence can occur in a woman is due to a prolapse (or protrusion) of either the bladder or the uterus through the vaginal opening. It is recommended to see a urologist for an internal exam. A suspension of the bladder done by surgery can make all the difference in the world for some patients.

- Products such as D-Mannose, cranberry pills and AZO help lower the acidity of the urine.
- Drink plenty of liquids to help wash out the bacteria.
- Avoid caffeinated or carbonated drinks as they can irritate the bladder
- Urinate often and try to empty the bladder completely
- Change sanitary pads often
- Always wipe front to back
- Keep the penis and vaginal area clean: for a male, using a maxi pad in the under garment to wick urine away from the penis can make changes easier. Also, the buttock skin is better protected from urine.

If you have a foley catheter:

A foley catheter is a tube inserted through the urethra of a male or female into the bladder. It stays being secured at the neck of the bladder by a balloon at the tip of the catheter. The balloon is inflated through a small Y valve at the other end of the catheter. The foley catheter is then attached to a urinary drainage bag, which collects the urine. It is important to empty the bag when half full so it does not begin to leak. There are calibrations on the bag so you can measure the drainage. The usual drainage amount should be around 2000 cc (milliliters) in 24 hours. Keeping a stabilizer device on the leg helps the catheter not to be pulled.

Foley catheters do not come without their own set of problems. Any invasive device in the body such as a catheter can cause infections. It is important to drink large amounts of fluids to keep the tubing patent and flowing. You may see some mucus, or specks of blood in the tube. It is when the urine goes from yellow to red, that something more serious is going on. Bladder spasms can also occur, causing some leakage of urine.

Patients with foley catheters usually have a visiting nurse who visits monthly to change the catheter, and more frequently to irrigate it if it is blocked for some reason. By calling the agency assigned, the nurse would come out and use sterile water to flush out the catheter to get it draining again. If there is no urine in the bag for over 4-8 hours, the visiting nurse should be called.

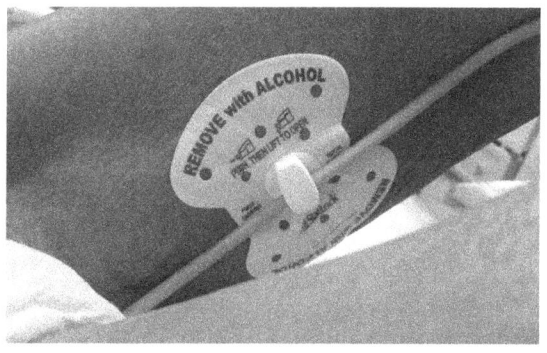

Catheter stabilizer

Care of a foley catheter:

- Always wash your hands before and after touching the catheter
- Check the area around the exit site of the catheter for inflammation or signs of infection. Signs of infection include irritated, swollen, red, tender skin or pus around the catheter exit site.
- Do not apply powder or lotion to the skin around the catheter

When you have a foley catheter, it is important to know that it is inserted by a nurse using sterile technique. The tubing and bag need to be connected to it carefully to maintain a closed system. The foley bag needs to stay below the person's body, then hooked it to a hospital bed rail, and not placed on the floor.

If the person is in a wheelchair, be sure to secure the drainage bag using the clip on the tubing above it, and attach it to the lower part of the back of the wheelchair. When turning someone in bed, always remember about the catheter and that it needs to be unclipped from the bed frame, and placed on the bed, moving with the patient to prevent it from being yanked. If there is leakage of urine around the exit site of the catheter or you notice little urine in the bag, then the catheter balloon might be deflating.

If the person is able to walk, the "night urinary drainage bag" is changed to a leg bag for day use. If the urinary drainage bag needs to be changed to a leg bag you will need:

- A pair of gloves
- Alcohol wipe
- Cap to apply to the tube that is disconnected

First, wash your hands and apply gloves

- Open the alcohol pad
- Gently screw off the tubing at the attachment site above the rubber port
- Wipe the alcohol pad on the white cone tip of the leg bag tubing
- Gently screw the new tubing into the Foley catheter
- Strap the leg bag to the leg

Acute Urinary Retention

This is a common problem in the older male. Think of the prostate gland like a donut with a straw (the urethra) running through the center. If the gland gets enlarged, the opening gets smaller and squeezes on the urethra (the straw). The "straw" gets squeezed, and urine gets trapped above the prostate gland with little to no urine getting through. You get the feeling you still need to void, but no urine comes out.

Unfortunately, if you have these symptoms going to the ER is necessary. The urine will be tested for signs of UTI. A catheter will be inserted to empty the bladder and see how much urine was retained. Sometimes, over 1000 cc of urine can come out very quickly.

Sometimes urinary retention happens from some medications. Benadryl is one such medication that is found in allergy medications and is used to help with sleep. Other medications are calcium channel blockers and pseudoephedrine. For the older adult, all medications taken should be reviewed to make sure they do not cause reactions such as this.

A foley catheter may need to be left in place, and the person has to go home from the hospital with it. A visiting nurse will be ordered to keep an eye on things at home and make sure the caregiver knows how to take care of the catheter. If the urologist wants to have the catheter removed, the nurse will remove it, then watch that the person is urinating and how much. If there is no urine in 8 hours, the person either needs to go back to the hospital, or the catheter needs to be reinserted.

Benign Prostatic Hypertrophy or Hyperplasia (BPH)

This condition is a noncancerous enlargement of the prostate gland and becomes common as most men age. The symptoms include frequent urination, trouble starting to urinate, a weak stream, inability to urinate, getting up at night to urinate, or loss of bladder control. If urine continues to back up into the bladder, urinary tract infections can occur. UTIs are less common, but more serious when they happen to a male. In addition, kidney stones and chronic kidney disease can ensue.

It is not clear how BPH happens. Family history can be one risk factor, along with obesity, type 2 diabetes, and erectile dysfunction. More than half of males over the age of 50 have BPH. Some things to do to reduce mild symptoms is to lose weight, exercise and decrease caffeine intake. If symptoms are more significant, alpha blockers such as Terazosin or 5 alpha -reductive inhibitors, finasteride, is ordered by your HCP or urologist.

Vaccines

According to the Centers for Disease Control (CDC), Pneumonia is one of the most common and deadliest diseases that can plague the older or disabled bedbound or frail person.

CDC recommends PCV15 or PCV20 for adults who never received a PCV and are:

Ages 65 years or older
Ages 19 through 64 years old with certain risk conditions

If PCV15 is used, it should be followed by a dose of PPSV23.

Adults who received an earlier PCV (PCV7 or PCV13) should talk with a vaccine provider. The provider can explain available options to complete the pneumococcal vaccine series.

Adults 65 years or older have the option to get PCV20 if they have already received PCV 13 (but not PCV15 or PCV20) at any age
AND
PPSV23 at or after the age of 65 years old

The pneumococcal vaccine is also recommended for people with chronic illnesses such as diabetes, lung diseases such as emphysema, asthma, alcoholism, chronic heart, and liver disease, weakened immune systems like cancers, or absent spleen. Also, smokers are recommended to get it.

You can get a flu vaccine in one arm and at the same time, get the pneumococcal vaccine in the other. You may want to take a Tylenol later in the day If you are not feeling well. The side effects of the pneumonia vaccine can include fever, loss of appetite, fatigue, headache, and redness at the injection site. The PPSV23 can also cause redness at the injection site, fever, and muscle aches. Symptoms can last up to two days. It is good to write this information in you Mom's log book for your records.

Another important vaccine that is recommended for adults aged 50 or older is the SHINGRIX (Shingles) vaccine or RZV, which stands for recombinant zoster vaccine. Shingrix had replaced Zostavax vaccine as of November 1, 2023 as the preferred vaccine to prevent shingles (herpes zoster). Adults 19 years and older who have or will have a weakened immune system should also consider getting this vaccine. The shingles vaccine is not given to someone over 80 because its effects diminish with age. Check with your HCP if there are any drugs you take that may have to be temporarily stopped, such as prednisone, cyclosporine, cancer chemotherapy and anti-viral drugs. These drugs are known to interfere with the action of the vaccine.

Possible side effects from this vaccine are Guillain-Barre syndrome, pain, redness, and swelling at the injection site. You can also get shivering, headache, fever and fatigue. The CDC recommends two doses of Shingrix vaccine, separated by 2-6 months. According to the CDC, the vaccine has been found to be effective for up to 10 years and is unlikely at this time, that booster shots will be needed.

It is to be given regardless of past episode of herpes zoster or having received the live zoster vaccine (ZVL) or Zostavax in the past. The vaccine should be given greater than 2 months after the ZVL was given. This vaccine is covered by Medicare.

Tetanus, diphtheria, and pertussis (Tdap) is a recommended vaccine by the CDC for adults to get every 10 years. Tetanus, sometimes called "lockjaw" is caused by bacteria found in the soil, dust, and manure. It can enter the body through a deep cut or burn. Diphtheria is a serious illness that can affect the tonsils, throat, nose, or skin. It can spread from person to person. Pertussis, also known as whooping cough, causes uncontrollable, violent coughing fits that make it hard to breathe. It can spread from person to person. Medicare Part D covers this vaccine.

For further information, go to www.CDC.gov to check on vaccine coverage.

Vaginal Yeast Infection

It is caused by too many yeast cells in the vagina. It is common in women of all ages, but especially those with diabetes, those who wear tight garments, or recently have been on antibiotics or steroids. The symptoms include itching, vaginal discharge, and irritation. Most infections get better on their own in 2 to 3 days. Treatment is usually a single dose of antifungal medication, such as Monistat. It can be purchased over the counter.

- Change undergarments regularly and wear cotton
- Do not scratch the area
- Use cool compresses to relieve the itch
- Wash the vaginal area daily with plain water/ mild soap and pat dry
- Wear loose-fitting clothes

When We Reach the End of Our Lives-

How can we stay home and die in our own bed? There is a process when we are born, and there is a process when we die. One of my patients lived with her son. He told me that as she was lying unconscious in her bed, he told her that it was alright to leave him and that she was in a beautiful dress, and her soldier (her husband) was waiting for her. A few minutes later, she passed, smiling.

Many of my patients died at home in their beds when I took care of them as their house calls clinician. When we start seeing changes in the person- weight loss, change in mental status, recurrent infections like pneumonia or urinary tract infections, uncontrollable fluctuations in blood sugars, development of spontaneous pressure injuries, frequent hospitalizations- we are aware that the body is deteriorating, and the person is moving to the next stage of life.

This is the time I discuss alternative care for a patient. Some children do not want their mother to die at home, and prefer to send her to the hospital where she may be evaluated there by hospice. She could then be transferred to a hospice residence or nursing home where hospice care is given. The person who does want to stay home will require more help with personal care, feeding and daily needs. Sometimes the children take turns moving in for weeks at a time. Some family members help by providing finances to pay for a live-in aide. It is important to think ahead and avoid a family crisis when your loved one gets terminally ill.

Unfortunately, an older person's condition can change quickly. This is when major decisions have to be made. Was she feeding herself, walking, watching TV and conversing with the aide; or has she been bedridden, incontinent, hand fed, and no longer recognizing her children? Sometimes, it takes a little while for the family to come to grips with the next step. Sometimes the family is all in agreement at the same time, but sometimes they are not.

This is where having a health care proxy in place is imperative. While the person was lucid, he would decide who would make medical decisions for him when he no longer can. There is an alternate proxy assigned as well. The witnesses who sign the form as well, need to be over 18, and not one of the proxies.

Sometimes, the family does not want hospice. We have to educate them that if the person's condition changes, they can call 911 and the paramedics will come to the home to determine her status. If she were to pass, the medical examiner needs to be called to assure there was not a suspicious reason for death, (since the patient is not on hospice). All deaths on hospice are also reported to the medical examiner. The nurse practitioner is then notified to complete the death certificate (in the state of NY). The practicing guidelines for a nurse practitioner vary from state to state.

Palliative care is how most home programs are done until hospice is determined. The patient has a life expectancy of 2 years. The goal is to enhance the quality of life by providing medical, spiritual, nursing and psychosocial intervention. This care can help patients experience peace, comfort, and dignity. Support services such as physical therapy and aide services can help with day-to-day care.

The hospice program was first started in Great Britain and now is in countries all over the world. When a referral is made to hospice, the intake coordinator speaks with the HCP about why he thinks his patient should be referred to the program. The hospice team will follow up with all referrals who do not get admitted to hospice. Hospice can be called out at a later time.

It is important to know that when agreeing to hospice, blood work, urine tests, x-rays, and hospitalizations cease. This is because the patient is no longer receiving aggressive treatment aimed at curing illness; rather they are receiving supportive treatment aimed at symptom management and keeping the patient as comfortable as possible. If the family should bring the patient to the hospital to seek aggressive treatment, they will need to revoke their hospice benefit, or they will be responsible for hospital costs.

Patients are evaluated by the hospice nurse regularly to manage the patient's symptoms, and see if they meet the criteria to remain on hospice. Patients can "graduate" from hospice after a year's time because their condition improved, not worsened. Another interesting finding is many of the medications the patient was taking, Aricept, Lipitor, Calcium, Vitamin D, etc. are stopped when hospice begins because they are no longer considered necessary. Sometimes the person feels better when some medications are stopped.

When the hospice program starts, a comfort kit. The kit consists of mostly liquid or sublingual (under the tongue) medications for pain, shortness of breath, nausea, constipation, fever and restlessness. These are emergency medications that may be needed and should only be given as directed by the hospice nurse. Oxygen, a hospital bed, Hoyer lift (if appropriate), overbed table, wheelchair, and other equipment may be delivered. The hospice nurse reviews with the private aide and family members how to administer medications.

Music and massage therapy, ongoing bereavement for the family, spiritual support, home health aides, and support by social workers are all part of the program. Specialty consults are available in certain instances. Hospice staff is on call 24 hours a day and can be called to deal with any problem or concern. This program helps the family feel like they have the support every minute of the day. Most insurance carriers cover hospice care.

There are some common misconceptions about hospice. Some clinicians and family think that when a person is placed on hospice:

- They can never get off the program
- That everyone has "given up" on the person's medical care

- You need a referral from your clinician
- The patient has to give up all his medications and take morphine
- You have to be homebound to be on hospice
- Hospice ends at the time of death
- The patient cannot go to the ER for any reason
- Concurrent care is accessible for children but not for adults

To help dispel the above myths, hospice lasts for 14 months after the person dies where family gets support and outreach letters. The person can decide to cancel hospice at any time. Anyone can make a referral to hospice; it does not have to be your HCP. The patient is in control and can decide not to stop any of their medications. If the person needs sutures or a procedure, he will be allowed to go to the ER for care. Adults can have more than one clinician while on hospice.

There are phases that the patient goes through during the process of dying. First is the change in her breathing pattern as it becomes more erratic, and with gurgling sounds. Mottling or color changes on the soles of the feet, and loss of consciousness are indications that the time is nearing.

If your loved one were to pass, the family is to call hospice first, and the hospice nurse will come to the home to pronounce her. The funeral home is then notified to take care of everything. In NY, the nurse practitioner could be the hospice attending clinician and will be responsible to complete the death certificate. Otherwise, the medical director or HCP would be responsible.

When your loved one has passed, you will go through the five stages of grief.

A Quick Story-

When we heard that Steve's mom was brain dead from a ruptured aneurysm while visiting her son in Bethlehem, PA, Steve as the HCP and I packed up some belongings for a 3 – hour drive to St. Luke's Hospital ER.

The doctor was relieved to know Steve had the HCP papers as his mom was on a respirator when we arrived. The doctor said Mary had no brain waves and that the respirator was keeping her alive.

The chaplain was called to anoint her and to pray with us. The respirator was then unplugged and removed from the room. Over the next 15 minutes we stayed with Mom- Steve was at her head and I was at the foot of the bed.

As mom took her last breath, the room lit up and I could feel light touches all over me. I began to smile and giggle. I knew, then, that Mary, a devoted Christian, was being carried by all of God's angels to heaven, and I was probably being touched by their wings!

Revelation 21:4 *He will wipe away every tear from their eyes, and death shall be no more, neither shall there be mourning nor crying, nor pain anymore, for the former things have passed away.*

(Go to the National Institute on Aging Website for Advanced Care Planning information/ forms).

The Five Stages of Grief

by Elisabeth Kubler Ross & David Kessler

1. DENIAL

These stages do not last for months but last for minutes as you move from one to the other and sometimes back again to other stages.

This is the first of the five stages of grief. Life makes no sense, and you are in a state of shock or denial. At this time, you find a way to just get through the day. It is a way of letting in only as much as you can handle. Beginning the acceptance by asking "why", you are unknowingly beginning the healing process. All the feelings that you were denying are now starting to come out.

2. ANGER

Anger is the second of the five stages of grief. You need to be willing to feel your anger. It is a time you feel deserted or abandoned. You may show anger to your friends whose spouses are still here, or your doctor, or even God if you believe. You may be angry at someone who did not come to the funeral or someone who did not have time for you when you needed it. Under the anger is your pain. The anger is just another way of showing how much you loved.

3. BARGAINING

This stage is when we ask God to reverse what happened to your loved one- "I wish we found the tumor earlier." If only..... causes you to find fault in ourselves and that we could have done something differently.

4. DEPRESSION

This stage comes after bargaining when our attention is moved right into the present. Grief enters our lives on a deeper level than you could ever imagine. It is important to know that depression is not a sign of mental illness. "Depression is actually an appropriate response to a great loss." We wonder if life is worth living, and why go on? It is unusual to not feel depressed after losing someone close. The loss settles deep in your soul, and you begin to realize he or she is not coming back. "If grief is a process of healing, then depression is one of the many necessary steps along the way."

5. ACCEPTANCE

Acceptance is not to be confused with "everything is OK." Most people never feel OK about losing someone they love. This stage is about accepting that the person is physically gone from your world as you know it. We never will like this reality, but it is now the new norm, and so we accept it. Our roles may be re-assigned, or we take them on. There will be good and bad days. We never replace what's lost, but we make new connections with others and begin to live life again. The stages of grief need to be given its time.

Https://grief.com is a great website that has a list of organizations and sites to help with grief. Consider calling your church or place of worship; or hospice for bereavement group information near you.

https://www.griefrecoverystartshere.com

https://drugfree.org/article/grief-resources-for-families/

Because love never dies

What is Ambiguous Loss?

Ambiguous loss is a type of grief that occurs when there is no clear end resolution to an ongoing situation. Pauline Boss PhD, a leading therapist in family stress, coined the phrase "ambiguous loss" back in the 1970's.

There are two types:

1. A person has a profound sense of loss and sadness that is **not** associated with a death of a loved one. You grieve for the person who is alive but is emotionally or relationally no longer part of your life, as in divorce, estrangement, incarceration, a chronic illness like dementia, or relocation to a new country.

   In this book, we are talking about the caregiver. The caregiver is caring for someone who is physically there but no longer psychologically present. There may be times when the person had some lucidity, like being his old self, but then becomes absent again. This caregiver could simultaneously experience the second type of ambiguous loss, such as divorce, etc.

2. When a loved one is physically absent, you do not know if they are dead or alive but they remain in your thoughts i.e. an estranged child, missing person, addiction that leads to abandonment. In these situations, a formal good bye does not happen which leads to a lack of closure.

   The goal is to help with resilience for the person to live with the loss, even though it does not resolve. His/her grief could "freeze" since they do not get a chance to let grief run a normal course.

Tips for coping with ambiguous loss:

- Name what you are going through
- Work towards acceptance, which isn't the same as closure
- Reach out for support- stay socially connected
- Look for silver linings – the good in your memories
- Get involved in a cause
- Be kind to yourself

Cognitive Behavioral Therapy and Acceptance Cognitive Therapy are two types of therapy that focus on mindfulness as coping skills.

Treat it by using "both-and" instead of "either-or"; example: "George is still here and also is gone".

(Mayo Clinic Health System April 10, 2023)
"Ambiguous Loss: Learning to Live with Unresolved Grief" by Pauline Boss PhD

Moving on.... the next chapter for the caregiver

It has been over a year since Axel has died. The first few months, Jynx saw her friends and just took the time to think about all the years of caring for Axel. She did attend grief counseling for family members who cared for someone who died from Alzheimer's disease. She went to the gym, took a stained-glass class, and traveled to visit her grown children who live in other states. She also caught up on her medical care: mammogram, Moh's biopsy of a lesion on her nose, a hip replacement that was way overdue.

My friend, Jynx said that at the funeral for her husband, someone said to her "what are you going to do now?" She said all she knew for the last 10 years was how to be a caregiver, today she said is "the first day I lost my full-time job." I can bet it is hard to go back to who you were before a caregiver because it takes so much out of the person. Everything about their life is on hold while they are caring for others.

One year later, she was ready to go through the house of 30 years and begin to purge anything that could be discarded. Her children came and took the tools, a car in the garage, and old memorabilia from their college days. I became close with Jynx as she went through the stages of grief. I was helping her pack up the other day, and she came across a basket of old love letters from Axel. It was time for me to leave her with her memories; all a part of healing and to move on. She found a 2-bedroom condo in a senior-gated community. She is moving to Texas to be closer with her son and his wife now expecting their third child. Her daughter is expecting her first child and lives overseas.

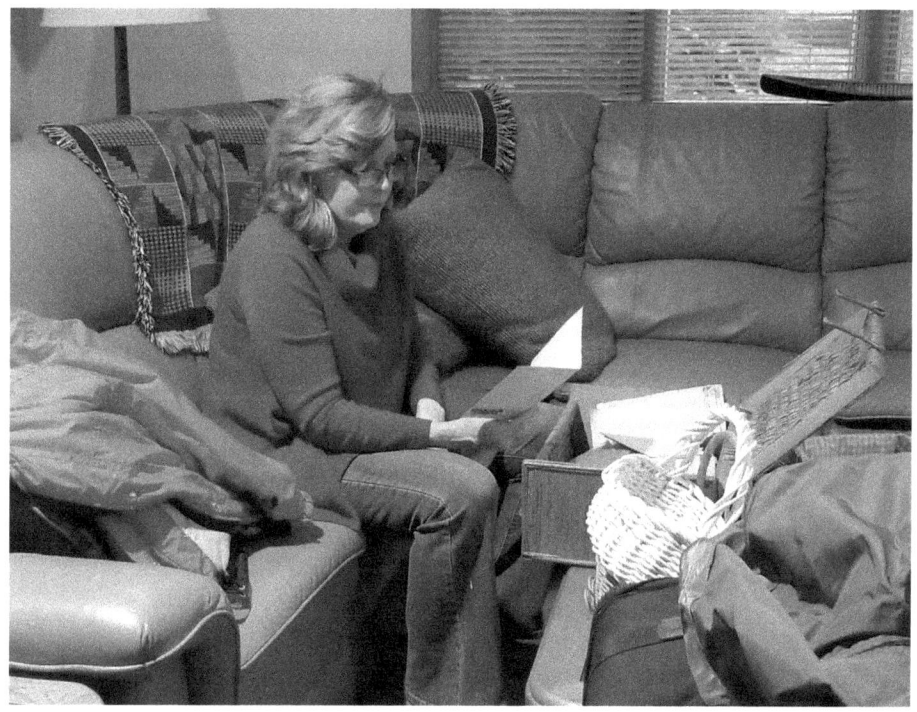

One of my patient's named Winni died. She was a poet. Her husband gave me a book of their love poetry to each other, with pictures of Winni throughout the book. This was Tom's way of working through his grief of loss. He shared something with me that was very close to his heart, and I will cherish the book always.

I took care of a 90-year-old woman whose daughter lived with her. She turned the living room into a bedroom for her mother: hospital bed, organizing shelves filled with undergarments, cleaning agents, medications and the like. The daughter quit her job working in a lab to care for her mother. She was single and had no children. Her life revolved around her mother. She rarely received medical care for herself or got out to get her hair cut or see friends. When her mother died years later, she bought a new couch, had the living room painted, and was lucky enough (because she stayed in touch with her friends at the lab) to get her job back.

Epilogue

We have no idea how long our "dash" is so live every moment and day as if its your last. We will have our reprieves of being a full-time caregiver but we will always be a caregiver to someone. Remember to be kind to yourself, and find your purpose God has meant for you. I found mine and I am always learning.

I hope you found this book helpful as your place to find medical tips and tools. Remember, thanks to you, your family member had less stress and hospital admissions……wouldn't that be good for you when you need it someday? We all hope and pray to grow old without a medical crisis.

Please pass this information on.

Romans 8:28 And we know that in all things
God works for the good of those who love him,
who have been called according to his purpose.

The Glossary

- 72 Decisions in 72 hours- a guide to follow after the death of a loved one

- Mini-Mental State Exam- A practical method for grading the cognitive state of patients

- Patient Health Questionnaire -9 Depression Screen scoring guide

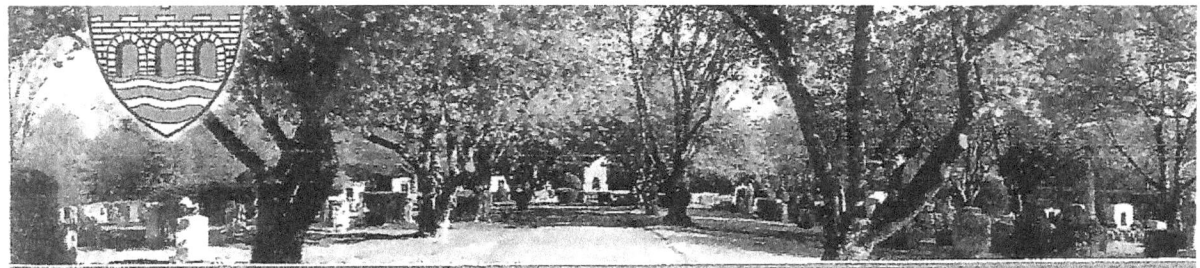

When a loved one passes, there are many decisions to make in a short period of time. Use this list to start your own burial planning and share it with your family.

72 DECISIONS IN 72 HOURS

1. Consult your cemetery Family Advisor for information
2. Name, address and telephone numbers
3. How long at present address
4. Date of birth
5. Place of birth
6. Legal proof of age or birth certificate
7. Citizenship, citizenship papers
8. Social Security Number
9. Business name or employer's address/contact
10. Father's name
11. Father's birthplace
12. Mother's maiden name
13. Mother's birthplace
14. Military Service Serial Number (if applicable)
15. Military Discharge Certificate (if applicable)
16. Legal Will and Power of Attorney
17. Pensions
18. Insurance Policies (life, health, car, property)
19. Investments
20. Bank books, account numbers
21. Deeds to properties (house, cottage)
22. Income tax returns, receipts, cancelled checks
23. Disability claims
24. Cemetery Certificate of Ownership
25. Marriage License
26. Addresses of children, relatives, close friends, etc.
27. Passwords: computer, accounts, social media
28. Meet with funeral director, cemetery advisor and/or clergy about details
29. Choose cremation or burial
30. Select style of urn or casket
31. Place where service is to be held. (e.g. funeral home; parish)
32. Reception location (funeral home, church, other)
33. Service type (religious, military, casual, themed, etc.)
34. Celebrant (funeral director, clergy, other)
35. Choose flowers and/or a commemorative display
36. Choose music (spiritual, popular, live or recorded)
37. Select readings (religious and/or secular)
38. Charitable organizations for in memoriam donations
39. Select the cemetery/mausoleum (niche or crypt location)
40. Vault or sectional crypt
41. Style of memorial (marker, stone, niche, bench, etc.)
42. Decorative elements and inscriptions
43. Interment service details, celebrant, etc.
44. Note the details/people to be included in obituary
45. Make notes on what to include in eulogy
46. Transportation for deceased, family
47. Determine budget and how expenses will be paid: (Full amount due at the time of crisis, or, in affordable installments available by pre-planning) Who to notify when death occurs:
48. Funeral home and cemetery
49. Doctors/medical practitioners
50. Notify relatives, friends, colleagues, neighbors
51. Insurance agents (life, health and accident)
52. Organizations (religious, fraternal, civic, veterans, unions)
53. Lawyer, accountant and executor bankers, investors, creditors, government responsibilities at time of death:
54. Set time/date of services, visitation, interment
55. Clothing for the deceased
56. Create online memorial (e. g. Sharing Memories TM)
57. Social media announcements
58. Write eulogy or provide notes to assist the writer
59. Check and sign legal papers, burial permits, etc.
60. Place obituary or provide vital statistics about deceased to newspaper
61. Arrange lodging for out-of-town guests
62. Make list of callers and floral tributes for mailing thank you cards
63. Arrange for any special religious requirements
64. Check Will regarding specific wishes
65. Order the Death Certificate
66. Arrangements for care of dependents and pets
67. Arrange clergy participation, pay clergy fees
68. Pay utilities and other current or urgent bills (mortgage or rent, taxes, installment payments)
69. Pay any outstanding medical or legal fees
70. Pay florist and caterers, unless paid in advance
71. Pay funeral fees, unless paid in advance
72. Pay cemetery fees, unless paid in advance

(Information provided by Arbor Memorial – Toronto, Canada)

The Mini-Mental State Exam

Patient _____ Examiner _____ Date _____

Maximum	Score	
		Orientation
5	( )	What is the (year) (season) (date) (day) (month)?
5	( )	Where are we (state) (country) (town) (hospital) (floor)?
		Registration
3	( )	Name 3 objects: 1 second to say each. Then ask the patient all 3 after you have said them. Give 1 point for each correct answer. Then repeat them until he/she learns all 3. Count trials and record. Trials _____
		Attention and Calculation
5	( )	Serial 7's. 1 point for each correct answer. Stop after 5 answers. Alternatively spell "world" backward.
		Recall
3	( )	Ask for the 3 objects repeated above. Give 1 point for each correct answer.
		Language
2	( )	Name a pencil and watch.
1	( )	Repeat the following "No ifs, ands, or buts"
3	( )	Follow a 3-stage command: "Take a paper in your hand, fold it in half, and put it on the floor."
1	( )	Read and obey the following: CLOSE YOUR EYES
1	( )	Write a sentence.
1	( )	Copy the design shown.

_____ Total Score

ASSESS level of consciousness along a continuum _____

Alert Drowsy Stupor Coma

"MINI-MENTAL STATE." A PRACTICAL METHOD FOR GRADING THE COGNITIVE STATE OF PATIENTS FOR THE CLINICIAN. *Journal of Psychiatric Research*, 12(3): 189-198, 1975. Used by permission.

PATIENT HEALTH QUESTIONNAIRE-9
(PHQ-9)

Over the last 2 weeks, how often have you been bothered by any of the following problems? (Use "✔" to indicate your answer)	Not at all	Several days	More than half the days	Nearly every day
1. Little interest or pleasure in doing things	0	1	2	3
2. Feeling down, depressed, or hopeless	0	1	2	3
3. Trouble falling or staying asleep, or sleeping too much	0	1	2	3
4. Feeling tired or having little energy	0	1	2	3
5. Poor appetite or overeating	0	1	2	3
6. Feeling bad about yourself — or that you are a failure or have let yourself or your family down	0	1	2	3
7. Trouble concentrating on things, such as reading the newspaper or watching television	0	1	2	3
8. Moving or speaking so slowly that other people could have noticed? Or the opposite — being so fidgety or restless that you have been moving around a lot more than usual	0	1	2	3
9. Thoughts that you would be better off dead or of hurting yourself in some way	0	1	2	3

FOR OFFICE CODING _0_ + _____ + _____ + _____

=Total Score: _____

If you checked off any problems, how difficult have these problems made it for you to do your work, take care of things at home, or get along with other people?

Not difficult at all	Somewhat difficult	Very difficult	Extremely difficult
☐	☐	☐	☐

Developed by Drs. Robert L. Spitzer, Janet B.W. Williams, Kurt Kroenke and colleagues, with an educational grant from Pfizer Inc. No permission required to reproduce, translate, display or distribute.

www.ingramcontent.com/pod-product-compliance
Lightning Source LLC
LaVergne TN
LVHW070521070526
838199LV00072B/6670